Work and the Older Person
Increasing Longevity and Well-Being

Work and the Older Person

Increasing Longevity and Well-Being

EDITORS

Linda A. Hunt, PhD, OTR/L, FAOTA

Pacific University
Professor, School of Occupational Therapy
Director, Gerontology Program
Hillsboro, Oregon

Caroline Wolverson, DipCOT, DipHT, MSc

York St John University
Lord Mayor's Walk
York, United Kingdom

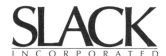

SLACK
INCORPORATED

www.Healio.com/books

ISBN: 978-1-61711-078-8

Copyright © 2015 by SLACK Incorporated

Cover photo reprinted with permission of Patrick Cote, Daily Inter Lake.

The procedures and practices described in this publication should be implemented in a manner consistent with the professional standards set for the circumstances that apply in each specific situation. Every effort has been made to confirm the accuracy of the information presented and to correctly relate generally accepted practices. The authors, editors, and publisher cannot accept responsibility for errors or exclusions or for the outcome of the material presented herein. There is no expressed or implied warranty of this book or information imparted by it. Care has been taken to ensure that drug selection and dosages are in accordance with currently accepted/recommended practice. Off-label uses of drugs may be discussed. Due to continuing research, changes in government policy and regulations, and various effects of drug reactions and interactions, it is recommended that the reader carefully review all materials and literature provided for each drug, especially those that are new or not frequently used. Some drugs or devices in this publication have clearance for use in a restricted research setting by the Food and Drug and Administration or FDA. Each professional should determine the FDA status of any drug or device prior to use in their practice.

Any review or mention of specific companies or products is not intended as an endorsement by the author or publisher.

SLACK Incorporated uses a review process to evaluate submitted material. Prior to publication, educators or clinicians provide important feedback on the content that we publish. We welcome feedback on this work.

Published by: SLACK Incorporated
                   6900 Grove Road
                   Thorofare, NJ 08086 USA
                   Telephone: 856-848-1000
                   Fax: 856-848-6091
                   www.slackbooks.com

Contact SLACK Incorporated for more information about other books in this field or about the availability of our books from distributors outside the United States.

Library of Congress Cataloging-in-Publication Data

Work and the older person : increasing longevity and wellbeing / editors, Linda A. Hunt, Caroline Wolverson.
    p. ; cm.
  Includes bibliographical references and index.
  ISBN 978-1-61711-078-8 (alk. paper)
  I. Hunt, Linda A., editor. II. Wolverson, Caroline, 1965- editor.
  [DNLM: 1. Aged. 2. Longevity. 3. Work--psychology. 4. Quality of Life--psychology. 5. Retirement--economics. WT 30]
  RA776.75
  613.2--dc23
                       2014026911

Printed in the United States of America.

Last digit is print number: 10   9   8   7   6   5   4   3   2   1

DEDICATION

This book is dedicated in memory of my mother, Bess Fine. She taught me how employment contributes to quality of life, self-esteem, and purposeful living. This book is also dedicated to David Hunt, my husband, and Erin Hunt, my daughter. They love, support, and understand me throughout it all.

Linda A. Hunt, PhD, OTR/L, FAOTA

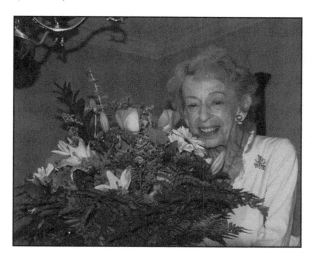

CONTENTS

About the Editors

Linda A. Hunt, PhD, OTR/L, FAOTA, is from St. Louis, Missouri and now lives in Oregon and Montana. She studies aging and directs the Graduate Certificate in Gerontology for Healthcare Professionals. In addition, she teaches a curriculum on aging and its impact on engagement in activities for occupational therapy programs at Pacific University and Chatham University. This book idea originated with Linda's love of older people, and the experiences of her mother, Bess Fine, who worked past age 70, and her aunt, Evelyn Myers, who volunteered past age 80. Both were role models for Linda. They inspired a work ethic. They taught her that engaging in work brings passion, purpose, and satisfaction to life.

Caroline Wolverson, DipCOT, DipHT, MSc, is from Yorkshire, England and is a senior lecturer in the Faculty of Health and Life Sciences at York St John University. She worked as an occupational therapist for 16 years in a variety of settings, and now teaches in the undergraduate occupational therapy program and masters-level Professional Health and Social Care studies.

Contributing Authors

Ross Andel, PhD (Chapter 8)
Associate Professor
School of Aging Studies
College of Behavioral and Community Sciences
University of South Florida
Tampa, Florida
International Clinical Research Center
St. Anne's University Hospital
Brno, Czech Republic

Marian Arbesman, PhD, OTR/L (Chapter 11)
Consultant, AOTA's Evidence-Based Practice
  Project
President, ArbesIdeas, Inc
Adjunct Assistant Professor
Department of Rehabilitation Science
University at Buffalo, State University of New
  York
Williamsville, New York

*Jane Cronin-Davis, PhD, MSc (Crim Psych),
  BHSc (Hons), BSc (Hons), BA, PGCAP,
  FHEA (Chapter 2)*
Head of Occupational Therapy Programme
Faculty of Health and Life Science
York St John University
Chair, College of Occupational Therapists
  Specialist Section Mental Health
Deputy Director Research Centre for
  Occupation and Mental Health
York, United Kingdom

Laura Dimmler, PhD, MHA (Chapter 10)
Professor of Healthcare Management
Pacific University
College of Health Professions
School of Healthcare Administration and
  Leadership
Master of Healthcare Administration Program
Hillsboro, Oregon

Erin E. Hunt, BS (Chapter 10)
Creative Director and Lead User Experience
  Designer
Forix Web Design
Portland, Oregon

Nancy E. Krusen, PhD, OTR/L (Chapter 5)
Associate Professor
School of Occupational Therapy
College of Health Professions
Pacific University
Hillsboro, Oregon

Susan Magasi, PhD (Chapter 4)
Assistant Professor
Department of Occupational Therapy
College of Applied Health Sciences
University of Illinois at Chicago
Chicago, Illinois

Denise M. Nepveux, PhD, OTR/L (Chapter 4)
Assistant Professor of Occupational Therapy
School of Health Professions and Education
Utica College
Utica, New York

Jeff Snodgrass, PhD, MPH, OTR/L (Chapter 7)
Area Chair & Program Director
Department of Occupational Therapy
Professor of Healthcare Administration &
  Occupational Therapy
Milligan College
Milligan College, Tennessee

Aimée Thompson, BSc (Hons) (Chapter 4)
Occupational Therapy Student
University of Illinois at Chicago
Department of Occupational Therapy
Chicago, Illinois

*Michael Wolverson, BA (Hons), BSc (Hons),
  MSC, RNMH, PGCE, RNT (Chapter 1)*
Lecturer in Learning Disability
Department of Health Sciences
University of York
York, United Kingdom

PREFACE

This is a book about aging, work, and the relationship between the two. This book is written by occupational therapists and others who are fascinated by aging and its impact on the desire to engage in occupations that are loved beyond what is traditional practice.

Throughout this book, older people have told us their stories. These stories, along with narratives from a range of sources, are used to support findings from research and illustrate the opportunities, challenges, frustrations, and choices that older people face in maintaining a productive lifestyle. This book is also a celebration of older people's continued passion for work.

It draws on a wide range of sources to provide a resource for decision makers, those providing employment to people working beyond traditional retirement age, and for those supporting people to remain in employment or find new employment. In addition, it can offer encouragement to those wishing to maintain a productive lifestyle beyond retirement age through the inspirational narratives contained in each chapter. Where requested, pseudonyms have been used for those telling their stories.

Finally, the book covers aging, current events, and the economy largely within Western societies. As countries struggle with the age of retirement and the consequent financial benefits paid to retirees, we hope to make an argument that working into old age, for many, actually contributes to longevity and greater quality of life.

Linda A. Hunt, PhD, OTR/L, FAOTA
Caroline Wolverson, DipCOT, DipHT, MSc

1

A Historical Perspective

Michael Wolverson, BA (Hons), BSc (Hons), MSC, RNMH, PGCE, RNT

The test of our progress is not whether we add more to the abundance of those who have much; it is whether we provide enough for those who have little.—Franklin D. Roosevelt (1937)

This chapter will offer an overview of the historical relationship between older people and work. In order to frame the historical context, it will broadly follow a sequential historical time line that begins before the Industrial Revolution in Europe and ends in the 21st century. There is consensus that the relationship between older people and work is extremely variable, depending on the cultural context in which this relationship takes place; however, this discussion will focus mainly on the relationship between older people and work within the historical and cultural context of Western Europe, North America, and other parts of the industrialized world, such as Australia. A key objective of the chapter is to demonstrate how cultural factors influenced and culminated in our modern views regarding older people and work.

HOW OLD WAS "OLD" IN THE PAST?

It is important to consider when a person is considered to be "old." Historical, sociological, and cultural factors have contributed to socially constructed perceptions of when a person is categorized as old. Thane (2000) lists the following factors that have been used to shape definitions of old:

- Chronologically by birth date
- Functionally in relation to fitness to accomplish certain tasks
- Biologically in relation to physical ability
- Culturally specific definitions and perceptions of old age

Hunt LA, Wolverson C.
Work and the Older Person: Increasing Longevity and Well-Being (pp 1-12).
© 2015 SLACK Incorporated.

At this point, it is useful to dispel a widely held belief that very few people in the preindustrial period lived to be "old" as gauged by contemporary longevity. Wrigley and Schofield (1989) have explained that this belief has been reinforced by measuring life expectancy from birth. It is indeed the case that life expectancy from birth in England between the 1540s and 1800 was approximately 35 years, but this was a consequence of high infant mortality lowering the average significantly. Thane has pointed out that those who survived infancy in early modern England had a good chance of reaching their late 40s and 50s, with many living considerably longer. Although the age at which people have been categorized as old fluctuates across time and cultures, there does seem to be consensus that the chronological age of 60 signifies the onset of old age. In ancient Greece, the obligation to perform military service ended at 60 (Finley, 1984). Similarly, since medieval times in England, 60 has been the age at which a person could acceptably withdraw from public activities. However, there have been differences in the definition of old age based on the type of work a person does. There are certain occupations and types of work in which the functional ability to work productively has resulted in the onset of old age being extended. Examples from early modern England include coroners, clergymen, members of the House of Lords, and the Aldermen who governed towns. Thane has stated that in the mid-17th century, the average age of death of Archbishops of Canterbury was 73. "This suggests that, at least among the 17th-century elite, people were not necessarily regarded as worn out or useless by this age" (Thane, 2000, p. 25). In direct contrast to this, and based on both a functional and biological interpretation of the onset of old age, those engaged in manual and physically demanding work were not expected to remain fully active in these roles much past the age of 50. Some respondents to the Royal Commission on the Poor Laws described male manual workers of 50 years of age as being old. Thus, it is evident that the diversification of and hierarchies of work have contributed to differences in the age at which a person has been considered to be old.

Definitions and the Historical and Cultural Context of Work

Grint (1998) has explored the historical and cultural context of work from a global sociological perspective and asserts that, to a large extent, work is both a social construct and a social product. He explains how powerful historical and sociological processes have resulted in the contemporary interpretation of the meaning and configuration of work in Western Europe and North America. Schooler, Caplan, and Oates (1998) have identified how four interlinking historical and cultural factors influence the social construction of older people and work as follows:

1. The specific economic and cultural events pertaining to the historical period in which an individual grows up

2. The ways in which older people themselves influence political decisions, the social norms and expectations within the societies they are aging in

3. The fact that political and economic changes that are developed in response to aging populations may not be sequential or orderly and can be reactive rather than proactive

4. The interaction between different age groups and other sub groups in society

In very broad terms, this consensual interpretation of work is that it is, at the very least, an expected component of an individual's life, if not a moral requirement of citizenship. In Western Europe and North America, a life span pattern has developed. Anderson (1985) has outlined what he described as the *modern life cycle*, which is an increasingly prolonged period in education that is designed to prepare people to engage in productive work. This is followed by a lengthy period of productive employment lasting approximately 40 years, but which in many Western countries became shorter between 1945 and 2008. Productive employment is then followed by a period of retirement, which until quite recently, often resulted in an abrupt withdrawal of the retired individual from productive employment. All countries that conform to this Westernized sociological model have arbitrary cut-off points based on the age when older people are expected or required to cease to be actively employed. This life span pattern has become the dominant and expected life course for the industrialized West; however, this status quo has not always existed, and arguably it has created a discriminatory system that makes it very difficult for older people to engage in employment. This, in turn, can result in stigmatization, marginalization, socially constructed dependency, and social exclusion. Indeed, Townsend (1981) and Macnicol (1998) have asserted that the constructed dependency of older people is largely a post-welfare state phenomenon, and one of the few forms of socially acceptable unemployment. This chapter will explore how this widely accepted life span pattern developed.

WORK AND THE OLDER PERSON IN PREINDUSTRIAL SOCIETIES

There are few narratives that relate to older people and work in preindustrial societies; however, one of the most famous is the Inquisition Register of Jacques Fournier, who compiled an extensive narrative history of the French village of Montaillou between 1318 and 1325 (Le Roy Ladurie, 1978). Le Roy Ladurie scrutinized the original, meticulously kept records of Fournier to produce a fascinating overview of the social mores, including the nature of work, that were prevalent in Europe in the early 14th century. Le Roy Ladurie's analysis of work in Montaillou indicates several themes, some of which still have resonance in contemporary society. It seems that there was no differentiation between older and younger people, and that expectations relating to work were the same for all adults, regardless of age. Achenbaum (2001) has discussed how this attitude of including all adults in the workforce to ensure the common good (or "commonwealth") was largely unchallenged until the late 19th century. Achenbaum also asserts that through both economic necessity and choice, older people have been expected to be productive throughout the majority of recorded history. A further factor illustrated by the testimonies of the people of Montaillou is that there was a relationship between religion and work, and that work was a moral imperative. The receipt of "alms" (charity) was also considered shameful. This attitude can be seen in the testimony of Emersend Marty of Montaillou, who said, "One does not acquire merit by giving alms to me, because I am capable of working" (Le Roy Ladurie, 1978, p. 340). Jean Maury, a resident of Montaillou, would only eat what he had produced himself, justified this by saying it was because "The Son of God said that man must live by the sweat of his brow" (p. 340). The testimonies of the people of Montaillou also indicate that although work was a moral obligation, people "worked to live" as opposed to living to work. Le Roy Ladurie paints something of an idyllic picture of the lives of the peasantry of Montaillou, with descriptions such as the following:

> The people of Montaillou were fond of having a nap, of taking life easy, of delousing one another in the sun or by the fire. Whenever they could, they tended to shorten the working day into a half day...At all events, work in itself was not a source of earthy consideration. For a peasant to farm his own land well was merely to show that he was not mad. The head of a household was expected to be a good neighbour, but not to kill himself with work. (Le Roy Ladurie, 1978, pp. 339-340)

This depiction of working to live is somewhat at variance with the Protestant work ethic that developed from Calvinistic beliefs in Northern Europe in the early 16th century and which will be discussed in depth later in the chapter.

The testimonies of the people of Montaillou provide one final perception of work, which is also reflected in contemporary interpretations of the meaning of work. The majority of workers were farmers who produced enough to live, and indeed, as stated by Jean Maury, "live by the sweat of their brow." Although this was largely the case, Montaillou was not an entirely subsistence economy. Subsistence economies have characterized preindustrial societies, and in essence, these economies produced barely enough to feed their population, with little or no surplus. In early 14th century Europe, most local economies regularly did produce a surplus, and this resulted in both a diversification and reinterpretation of work. As a consequence of Montaillou and the surrounding economy producing more than was required for subsistence, it was possible for a minority of the population to develop new types of work. This produced a philosophical dichotomy in relation to the meaning of work, which has echoes in the contemporary division of labor. This dichotomy was largely between work that involves manual and physical toil such as farming and working roles that are cerebral and sedentary and involve some degree of skill. In Montaillou, this caused some degree of resentment and anger based on the perception of what constituted work. Notable examples of this perception relate to the clergy, who were perceived to live off the labor of those doing "real" physical toil and to be undeserving of the rewards their work provided. Guillemette Argelliers of Montaillou stated that:

> The priests ought to live by the work of their own hands, according to the commandment of God, and not off the work of the people, as they do in fact. The priests, who expel people from the path of salvation, do all in order to be well dressed and well shod, in order to ride on horseback and eat well. (Le Roy Ladurie, 1978, p. 340)

It should be noted that there was far less resentment directed at those people who developed trades, such as comb making and tanning, because there appeared to be a more justified link between their efforts and reward. It is also the case that the clergy were enormously powerful at this time and could be seen to have control over their work, and this bred much resentment. Parallels can be drawn here in relation to older people and work in a contemporary context. Many people who are engaged in manual employment have little control over their working lives and are subject to arbitrary enforced retirement at an age when they are deemed no longer fit for physical work (Achenbaum, 2001). In addition, those who are perceived to live off the surplus of manual workers are not subject to enforced retirement ages and can work indefinitely. Societies develop hierarchies of work, and in Western societies, it is evident that in relation to certain categories of work, arbitrary retirement ages do not apply and older people carry on working within these roles. Examples of this phenomenon include politicians such as Winston Churchill, who in 1951 was elected Prime Minister of Great Britain at the age of 77, and Ronald Reagan, who was elected as the President of the United States for a second term at age 73. It should be noted that this was not exclusive to the 20th century, as the American President John Quincy Adams left the White House at age 61 in 1832, then went on to serve in Congress until he was 81. Pablo Picasso carried on working up to the day of his death at age 91, and the Rolling Stones, who were once icons of youthful rebellion, are still touring in their 70s.

Montaillou serves to illustrate how historical and cultural influences still have an impact on perceptions of work and the position of older people in relation to it. Economies that produce a surplus spawn a plethora of work roles and hierarchies that divide these roles into those that encourage or actively discourage older workers. This divide in the 21st century often is still as it was in Montaillou, with manual work that produces the surplus at the bottom of the hierarchy, and work that can only exist as a result of surplus valued more highly. Affluent modern industrial societies produce a huge surplus, and this has allowed for the development of relatively recent interpretations of the meaning of work. The great English social commentator George Orwell captured this dichotomy well in *The Road to Wigan Pier*:

> More than anyone else, perhaps, the miner can stand as the type of the manual worker, not only because his work is so exaggeratedly awful, but also because it is so vitally necessary and yet so remote from our experience, so invisible, as it were, that we are capable of forgetting it as we forget the blood in our veins. In a way it is even humiliating to watch coal miners working. It raises in you a momentary doubt about your own status as an 'intellectual' and a superior person generally. For it is brought home to you, at least while

you are watching, that it is only because miners sweat their guts out that superior persons can remain superior. You and I and the editor of the *Times Lit. Supp.,* and the Nancy poets and the Archbishop of Canterbury and Comrade X, author of *Marxism for Infants*—all of us *really* owe the comparative decency of our lives to poor drudges underground, blackened to the eyes, with their throats full of coal dust, driving their shovels forward with arms and belly muscles of steel. (Orwell, 1937, p. 31)

The discussion of the meaning of work in preindustrial societies outlined how certain categories of work were interpreted in a variety of philosophical and psychological ways. Furthermore, Orwell's comments indicate that industrialized economies allowed for the development of a vast array of ways in which people could be productively employed, and that there exists a socially constructed hierarchy of employment. This is an important consideration because it also indicates that employment is linked to social status and individual identity and that the concept of work is culturally variable. Philosophers since the ancient Greeks have endeavored to understand the nature of life and of work. There is a notion that work is, to some extent, an existential phenomenon. This is evidenced by the fact that some work, such as coal mining, can be seen as an economic necessity, whereas other forms of work, such as writing poetry, are perceived as cathartic indulgence. Many people who are independently wealthy, and for whom paid work is not a necessity, choose to continue to work. The existential issue in relation to work is basically that individuals have a range of options during their existence, and productive work is the preferred option of a majority. The eminent humanist philosopher Bertrand Russell, in *The Conquest of Happiness,* explores how work gives meaning to life, and along with aspects of existence, can lead to a happy life (1975). Alain de Botton has explored the contemporary meaning of work and how different occupations confer status and confirm an individual's identity in his books, *The Pleasures and Sorrows of Work* (2010) and *Status Anxiety* (2005). Having discussed a diverse range of productive employment, de Botton (2010) summarizes the common existential benefits of work thus:

> Our work will at least have distracted us, it will have provided a perfect bubble in which to invest our hopes for perfection, it will have focused our immeasurable anxieties on a few relatively small-scale and achievable goals, it will have given us a sense of mastery, it will have made us respectably tired, it will have put food on the table. It will have kept us out of greater trouble. (de Botton, 2010, p. 326)

It does appear that there is a consensus that productive work offers a great many individual benefits. Withdrawal from productive work, often as a result of arbitrary and enforced retirement ages, can abruptly rob older people of the benefits of work—their happiness, social status, and a large part of their identity.

THE PROTESTANT WORK ETHIC

In his book *Civilization: The Six Killer Apps of Western Power,* Niall Ferguson discusses the Protestant work ethic in relation to the predominance of the Western model of work. Ferguson (2011) explores how the Protestant work ethic has been a hugely influential component of the social construction of the perception of work across the industrialized Western world, and how this accounts for relative affluence within these cultures. The German sociologist Max Weber first used the term *Protestant ethic* after studying the evolution of work in Northern Europe and North America, from the Protestant Reformation of the early 16th century until the late 19th and early 20th centuries. In his seminal work, *The Protestant Ethic and the Spirit of Capitalism,* published in 1905, Weber succinctly outlined what has been the most widely accepted perception of work for almost 500 years across the Western world. He postulated that the Protestant Reformation in Northern Europe and the separation from the Catholic Church resulted in the Protestant work ethic. In very basic terms, the Protestant work ethic holds that work is an intrinsically virtuous activity and a moral imperative linked to Protestant Christian beliefs. Ferguson (2011) describes the characteristics of the Protestant work ethic in this way:

> Whereas other religions associated holiness with the renunciation of worldly things—monks in cloisters, hermits in caves—the Protestant sects saw industry and thrift as expressions of a new kind of hardworking godliness. The capitalist "calling" was, in other words, religious in origin. To attain...self-confidence [in one's membership of the Elect] intense worldly activity is recommended...[Thus] Christian asceticism...strode into the market place of life. "Tireless labour," as Weber called it, was the surest sign that you belonged to the Elect..."The Protestant ethic moreover, provided the capitalist with sober, conscientious, and unusually capable workers, who were devoted to work as the divinely willed purpose of life." For most of history, men had worked to live. But the Protestants lived to work. (Ferguson, 2011, pp. 261-262)

THE PROTESTANT WORK ETHIC, THE ELIZABETHAN POOR LAW, AND THE WORKHOUSE

The Elizabethan Poor Law and its enduring impact provides an excellent example of how the Protestant work ethic influenced the sociological and philosophical interpretation of work. It should be noted that although the Elizabethan Poor Law was enacted in England in 1601, the philosophies that underpinned it were evident across the northern countries of Europe that had undergone the Reformation, and subsequently North America after the colonization of its eastern seaboard by emigrants from these countries. It is of equal importance to note that the Poor Law influenced British social policy until the advent of the Welfare state in 1948. It codified the interpretation of work that was consistent with the Protestant work ethic, as outlined by Ferguson (2011). In relation to older people, the Elizabethan Poor Law reiterated the expectation that older people should work throughout the life span, if at all possible. The key components of the Elizabethan Poor Law were as follows (Thane, 2000):

- The "setting to work" of children whose parents could not maintain them and of adults who could not maintain themselves

- Local parishes being made responsible for providing assistance to the poor and "for the necessary relief of the lame, old, impotent, blind, and such other among them being poor and not able to work"

- Local parishes were to appoint "two or more substantial householders" to be overseers of the poor

- Local parishes were to collect a "compulsory poor rate" in order to distribute to the poor as "poor relief"

It is clear that provisions of the Elizabethan Poor Law were predicated on the belief that work was a moral imperative, dependency should be discouraged, and that all people, regardless of age, should work. To offset the cost of poor relief, those in receipt of it could be given work tasks, such as repairing roads, regardless of age. The original Elizabethan Poor Law of 1601 allowed for the provision of "out relief," whereby those in receipt of poor relief could remain at home. There was also some provision in the form of alms houses for those who could no longer live independently, and a piecemeal system of "houses of correction" and workhouses was developed. The belief that work is virtuous, and its corollary that dependency implies a moral failing, contributed to the notion of the "deserving" and the "undeserving poor." This division of the poor partially accounts for the Poor Law Amendment Act of 1834. Under this Act, poor relief was discouraged and workhouses became the main provision for dispensing poor relief. The workhouses were institutionalized settings with extremely strict regimes that were developed to deter the "undeserving poor." It was expected that only those in genuine need would be accommodated in them, and that inmates of the workhouses would work to subsidize the cost of their poor relief. The work that inmates were expected to do was often purposefully tedious. The working day was 10 hours long and tasks included milling corn, making sacks, unravelling lengths of rope, and crushing bones. Older inmates were expected to work at these tasks whenever possible (Thane, 2000). At the Liverpool workhouse, none of the inmates were exempt from work until they were 80 years of age. Older people who were considered not capable of much work and who were in receipt of some level of poor relief would still be expected to earn something. Thus, many older people combined some poor relief with an earned income. There are many meticulously kept parish and census records that illustrate this point. Thane has reported on a list of people in the Salisbury area in 1635 who could possibly combine poor relief with some amount of earned income. The list included:

> …a 90-year-old woman described as "lame in arm" who was earning sixpence per week supplemented by twelvepence poor relief…75-year-old widow Bagges, "lame in her hands", earned eightpence weekly and also received twelvepence relief. Walter Danyell, at age 81, earned 1 shilling per week supplemented by fourpence relief; his wife earned sixpence. Widow Harty earned sixpence at age 80 and received twopence relief. (Thane, 2000, pp. 91-92)

Records show that, wherever possible, the skills of older people that developed during their fully productive working lives were utilized for the common good. An example of this is provided by John Taylor of Maidstone, who had been a shoemaker until 1770, when he could no longer do this full time. The parish paid him to repair the shoes of the workhouse inmates, which he did until he died at age 80. James Carr, who was the parish coffin maker in Cowden, was admitted to the workhouse, but took his tools with him and continued to make coffins and engage in other carpentry tasks.

It is evident that efforts were consistently made to enable older people to remain as independent as possible, and that self-sufficiency was perceived to be a virtue. Sometimes, this was achieved by using poor relief to enable people to remain independent and productively engaged in work. For example, John Wells of Tonbridge was described as being old and infirm in 1768. Records show that the parish poor relief gave him sixpence to buy seeds and plant a vegetable plot. The fact that he didn't become a regular pensioner indicates that he must have been able to live off his plot and sell his produce in order to remain self-sufficient (Thane, 2000).

Boyer (2010) discussed regional variations in the numbers of older people seeking poor relief, but a consistently average estimate is approximately 26%. This indicates that a significant amount of older people either worked to support themselves or were supported by their families. Once again, records indicate that older people remained in productive work for as long as it was physically possible to do so. In many cases, older people would change working roles as a result of being physically unable to continue in their previous occupations. Older people who were unable to consistently work would take up part-time or casual roles. Mary Barker Read extensively explored this changing nature of work in five Kent parishes from 1662 to 1797. Read (1988) offers a vast list of casual work available to older people, including holding horses, sweeping up, fruit picking, hay making, collecting and selling herbs for medicines and flowers for posies, gathering and selling rushes for lighting, and cutting hazel for basket weaving. Many occupations were reserved for older workers who could no longer continue in their previous employment. These occupations were generally poorly paid and included watching prisoners, child minding, care-taking, serving in ale houses, and carrying goods.

Although older people were actively encouraged to engage in work to remain independent, when they were no longer capable of doing any work, they were treated benignly and provided for by either communities in which they lived or in the workhouses. In 1926 in Britain, 226,000 people were still accommodated in workhouses. Sutherland Ritch (2009) suggested that by this point the majority of older people in the workhouses were those in need of nursing care, and that there were well-intentioned attempts to respond to their needs.

THE PROTESTANT WORK ETHIC AND THE AMERICAN DREAM

The majority of the early settlers to the eastern seaboard of North America came from the Northern European countries that had undergone the Reformation, and their interpretation of work was based on the Protestant work ethic. In the very early 17th century, America was portrayed as a land of plenty with a cornucopia of riches. This depiction of the New World attracted emigrants from Northern Europe who were inculcated by the Protestant work ethic, and who understood that hard work would be a necessity if the continent's natural resources were to be harnessed. These early settlers and subsequent immigrants were also inspired to work in pursuit of the American Dream. In essence, the American Dream was the belief that wealth and contentment could be achieved by everyone who came to America, if only they worked hard enough. The American Dream has been one of the prevailing beliefs from the time of the Founding Fathers that still influences attitudes toward work, and perceptions of older people and work, in the 21st century. After the collapse of the Soviet Union in 1989, America was considered the only global superpower, and many observers believed that this status was achieved by a combination of the Protestant work ethic, the American Dream, and a surfeit of natural resources. It can be argued that America's global hegemony, and a perception that the Protestant work ethic and the American Dream create economic dynamism, have resulted in many other countries attempting to manage their economies based on these perceptions of work. Indeed, even the ostensibly communist Republic of China has developed a dynamic economy that now rivals America's. It would seem that the American model of work is now the dominant paradigm across the industrialized Western world, and this significantly influences the perceptions of older people and work.

The majority of the work undertaken by the early settlers to America's eastern seaboard involved working the land. Although written in the 18th century after the initial wave of settlement, Hector St. John de Crevecouer wrote of America:

> I do not mean, that everyone who comes here will grow rich in a little time; no, but he may procure an easy, decent maintenance by his industry. Instead of starving, he will be fed; instead of being idle, he will have employment; and these are riches enough for such men as come over here. (Cited in Achenbaum, 2001, p. 21)

There are clear echoes of the Protestant work ethic here. Subsequent social commentators, such as Benjamin Franklin, Thomas Jefferson, and Alexis de Tocqueville, have attributed the dynamism and success of America to the Protestant work ethic of the early settlers. They also reinforced the belief that all people, including older people, should work and contribute to the common good. Although working the land in a premechanized world could be extremely arduous, older people could still contribute to this process. The first federal census in America revealed that in 1790, 95% of the population were rural dwellers. In 1820, approximately three-quarters of all workers were farmers (Shover, 1976).

Achenbaum (2001) reports that documents from this time indicate that most older workers were farmers. He also explains that when older workers could no longer engage in physically demanding labor, such as plowing and clearing the land, they did other forms of agricultural work, such as shoeing horses. The experience and accumulated wisdom of older farm workers was perceived to be a valuable and productive contribution to the common good. That older people were expected to contribute their labor was also noticed by de Tocqueville, who observed that old age did not alter the expectation that people should remain productive. A combination of the American Dream and Protestant work ethic galvanized workers across the age range as they endeavored to not only better themselves, but also to create a dynamic and prosperous new nation. Achenbaum (2001) refers to this as a "…novus ordo seclorum—a new order of the ages—hinged on the ability of all age groups to remain productive, committed to working together for the benefit of all" (p. 23).

Foreign observers of American attitudes to work, such as the Oxford professor James Bryce, who had visited in 1888, commented consistently on how older workers were expected to remain productive in order to remain self-sufficient. America is a dynamic nation in which change is constant; however, the central beliefs that work is a moral imperative, hard work and effort will be rewarded by wealth and success, and that everyone should contribute to the common good remain dominant.

INDUSTRIALIZATION AND OLD AGE PENSIONS

The Industrial Revolution that began in Britain in the late 18th century, spreading across the countries of Northern Europe and North America, fundamentally changed the way that a majority of people have worked across the Western world (Hobsbawm, 1975). Subsequently, many other countries and cultures based on capitalist ideals developed some degree of industrialization. It has had a huge impact on working patterns, the relationship between people and work, and perceptions of those engaged in work.

Industrialization is characterized by the following:

- The mechanization of the means of extracting and managing natural resources
- The mechanization of the means of production
- The mass production of standardized products
- Innovation and constant refinement of the processes listed above
- Social change and urbanization
- The development of a proletariat
- Centralization of production
- Economies of scale and competition
- Maximization of worker efficiency and productivity
- Piecework

In his seminal work on the Industrial Revolution, Hobsbawm (1975) explained how the characteristics above significantly altered the nature of work. Hobsbawm, and later Macnicol (1998), also explored how these significant changes affected older workers. Britain was the cradle of the Industrial Revolution, and as such, is illustrative of how it affected older people and work. Prior to the Industrial Revolution, Britain was largely an agrarian economy, and older people could engage in productive work in agriculture long after they could no longer do physically demanding tasks. Before the Industrial Revolution, many of those not involved with agriculture were tradesmen. Others were involved in small-scale, unsophisticated cottage industries, which often involved working in their homes at such tasks as carding wool and spinning. Often, the raw materials would be delivered to the worker's home and the product collected later. Older people, mainly women, could engage in this productive work. The Industrial Revolution significantly changed this pattern. Rapid urbanization occurred as a result of people moving into towns, where they could find work in factories. Industrialization resulted in the concentration of manufacturing processes in large factories and other facilities that produced standardized products within economies of scale. First, this resulted in the demise of the cottage industries in which older people could remain productive. Second, industrialists demanded a reliable, physically fit workforce that could complete repetitive tasks quickly, particularly if they were involved in piecework. In many instances, this excluded older people from employment in the industrial system. Third, tradesmen, particularly if they were older, could not compete with factory production, and as a result, lost their livelihood. Macnicol (1998) summarized the cumulative effect of these changes on older workers, "industrialization creates a more specialized division of labor, with a greater premium on youth, skill and adaptability, and older people are seen as increasingly irrelevant to the labour process; Old age thus brings obsolescence" (p. 13).

Toward the latter part of the 19th century, it became increasingly clear that industrialists sought to employ younger workers while shedding older workers. Demographic changes also facilitated this process. In Europe, there was an increase in the birth rate, and this created a surfeit of available young and fit workers. In America, immigration created a workforce of young people in search of employment. In the later phases of the Industrial Revolution, increased mechanization and refinement of industrial processes resulted in the need for smaller workforces. Industrialization created competition both between industrial companies and between capitalist countries. Consequently, governments, businesses, and society in general became focused on ruthless efficiency, and young people were perceived to be more efficient than older workers. Hobsbawm (1975) comments, in relation to this unwillingness to employ older workers, that old age "…was a catastrophe to be stoically expected, a decline in earning power from the forties as physical strength ebbed—especially for the less skilled—followed by poverty, and like as not charity and poor relief" (p. 260).

This inadvertently contributed to what has become the modern life cycle of work, as many older people were forced to cease productive work, at or before the current age range of retirement, across the Western world. In order to manage this huge sociological change, the Western industrialized democracies introduced some level of state support for older people who were no longer working. Myles (1989) has discussed how Bismarck's Germany in the 1880s introduced old age pensions and other social benefits that later became the basic components of the "welfare state" across Western democracies. Other countries that introduced some degree of pension provision include the following:

- Denmark in 1891
- Austria in 1906
- Britain in 1908
- France in 1910
- The Netherlands in 1913
- Italy in 1919
- Belgium in 1924
- Canada in 1924
- The United States in 1935

It should be noted that the first old age pensions were far from generous. In Britain, where pensions would be paid initially at age 70, the Prime Minister, Lloyd George made it clear that "the five shilling pension was not intended to provide an income adequate for survival, but to supplement and to encourage saving and the support available from relatives and others" (Thane, 2000, p. 223).

CONCLUSION

The Industrial Revolution and the development of old age pensions not only resulted in the contemporary notion of the life cycle, but these fundamental, sociological changes significantly contributed to some of the negative beliefs about older people. Enforced retirement and the provision of pensions led to a belief that older people are unproductive, incapable of work, poor, in need of state subsidy, and a burden on productive taxpayers. Anderson (1985) and Myles (1989) discussed how the modern life cycle, particularly arbitrary retirement ages, has permeated cultural perceptions of older people in Westernized societies. This has led to a general acceptance of this system, resulting in older people being largely excluded from productive employment. From a historical and sociological perspective, this contemporary understanding of older people and productive employment has been a relatively recent phenomenon. This chapter has demonstrated that this modern perception of older people is, to some extent, a social construction, not an inevitability. It is becoming increasingly evident that demographic changes and the global recession that began with the collapse of Lehman Brothers in 2008 have already begun to influence the interface between older people and productive employment. The global recession has coincided with increasing longevity in the Westernized economies. Because of these huge financial and sociological changes, governments across the Western world have been forced to reconsider welfare provision and the provision of old age pensions. A majority of private sector companies no longer offer pension schemes, and public sector workers are being required to work longer before receiving their pensions. It is becoming increasingly evident that these factors have resulted in older people either being compelled or choosing to engage in productive employment for a longer period of time. Mechanisms such as the abolition of arbitrary retirement ages, phased retirement, and part-time and flexible hours have been put in place to enable older people to remain in productive employment. This may contribute to a positive reappraisal of old age. These new patterns of productive aging could reduce the stigma currently associated with old age, and lead to the improved social status of older people.

REFERENCES

Achenbaum, A. (2001). Productive aging in historical perspective. In N. Morrow-Howell, J. Hinterlong, & J. Sherraden (Eds.), *Productive aging: Concepts and challenges* (p. 21). Baltimore, MD: Johns Hopkins University Press.

Anderson, M. (1985). The emergence of the modern lifecycle in Britain. *Social History, 10*(1), 69-87.

Barker-Read, M. (1988). *The treatment of the aged poor in five selected west Kent parishes, from settlement to speenhamland, 1200-1800.* (Phd thesis, Open University 1988).

Boyer, G. R. (2010). *'Work for their prime, the workhouse for their age': A regional analysis of elderly pauperism in Victorian England.* Ithaca, NY: Cornell University.

de Botton, A. (2005). *Status anxiety.* London: Penguin Books.

de Botton, A. (2010). *The pleasures and sorrows of work.* London: Penguin Books.

Finley, M. (1984). The elderly in classical antiquity. *Aging and Society, 4*(4), 391-408.

Ferguson, N. (2011). *Civilization: The six killer apps of western power.* London: Penguin Books.

Grint, K. (1998). *The sociology of work* (2nd ed.). Cambridge: Polity Press.

Hobsbawm, E. J. (1975). *The age of capital: 1848-1875.* London: Abacus.

Le Roy Ladurie, E. (2008). *Montaillou: The promised land of error* (B. Bray, Trans.). New York: George Braziller. (Original work published 1978).

Macnicol, J. (1998). *The politics of retirement in Britain, 1878-1948.* Cambridge: Cambridge University Press.

Myles, J. (1989). *Old age in the welfare state: The political economy of public pensions.* Lawrence, KS: University Press of Kansas.

Orwell, G. (1937). *The road to Wigan pier.* London: Penguin Classics (reissue 2001).

Roosevelt, F. D. (1937, January 20). "One third of a nation": fdr's second inaugural address. Retrieved June 4, 2014, from http://historymatters.gmu.edu/d/5105/.

Russell, B. (1930). *The conquest of happiness.* New York: Liveright books (reissue 1999).

Schooler, C., Caplan, L., & Oates, G. (1998). Aging and work: An overview. In K.W. Schaie & C. Schooler (Eds.), *Impact of work on older individuals.* New York: Springer Publishing Company.

Shover, J. L. (1976). *First majority: The transforming of rural life in America.* DeKalb, IL: Northern Illinois University Press.

Sutherland Ritch, A. E. (2009). *Sick, aged and infirm: Adults in the new Birmingham workhouse, 1852–1912.* Birmingham, UK: University of Birmingham.

Thane, P. (2000). *Old age in English history.* Oxford: Oxford University Press.

Townsend, P. (1981). The structured dependency of the elderly: A creation of social policy in the twentieth century. *Ageing and Society, 1*(1), 5-28.

Weber, M. (2003). *The protestant work ethic and the spirit of capitalism* (T. Parsons, Trans.). Mineola, NY: Dover Publications. (Original work published 1905).

Wrigley, E. A., & Schofield, R. S. (1989). *The population history of England 1541-1871: A reconstruction.* Cambridge: Cambridge University Press.

2

An Occupational Science Perspective

Jane Cronin-Davis, PhD, MSc (Crim Psych), BHSc (Hons), BSc (Hons), BA, PGCAP, FHEA and Caroline Wolverson, DipCOT, DipHT, MSc

To business that we love we rise betimes, and go to't with delight.—William Shakespeare (1623)

This chapter will focus on work and the older person, and how occupational science might contribute to current considerations in this field. Occupational science has emerged as a discrete academic discipline that theoretically appreciates humans as occupational beings in the context of their own life worlds. It also seeks to investigate the interdependent relationship between occupation, health, and well-being; work being an occupation in its own right and an internationally recognized concept.

The discipline has much to offer when considering older people and their engagement and participation in personally constructed occupations. Occupations such as work have a financial impact, not only for the individual, but for the economic fabric of society. With the increasing aged population, there will be a need for older people to continue to make an economic contribution to their communities to help maintain a sustainable society.

Considering older people from an occupational perspective can contribute to and support healthy aging at both an individual and a societal level (Carlson, Clark, & Young, 1998). For the purposes of this chapter, concepts related to occupational science will be used to explore how people orchestrate their lives, and challenges and opportunities afforded by working into older age. Those of particular focus will be occupational deprivation, occupational alienation, occupational imbalance, and occupational disruption. This will be followed by exploration of occupational adaptation, occupational potential, and consideration of how these concepts enable us to view the positive contributions older people can make to a working environment and community.

Hunt LA, Wolverson C.
Work and the Older Person: Increasing Longevity and Well-Being (pp 13-23).
© 2015 SLACK Incorporated.

History and Development of Occupational Science

Occupational science was developed by academics at the University of Southern California, which implemented the now widely recognized doctoral program. The first paper published by Yerxa et al. (1989) introduced occupational science as a foundation for occupational therapy in the 21st century. This paper clearly defined this newly emerging academic discipline as "the study of the human as an occupational being including the need for and capacity to engage in and orchestrate daily occupations in the environment over the life span" (Yerxa et al., 1989, p. 6). It recognizes that humans are inherently complex, have an innate occupational nature, and that occupation itself is multifaceted (Molineux, 2010). Molineux (2010) emphasizes that as humans we have a need to engage in occupations in our environments, and in addition, the essential capacities to do so. Occupation has been defined in various ways by authors in the fields of both occupational science and occupational therapy. What best fits for the purposes of this chapter is the definition proposed by Townsend (1997): "All the active process of looking after ourselves and others, enjoying life, and being socially and economically productive over the life span and in various contexts" (p. 19).

Additionally, Molineux (2010) suggests that human occupation involves active engagement, is meaningful and purposeful, and is contextualized within multiple environments. A work place is one such environment that requires considerable engagement for successful and positive participation.

One of the seminal pieces of research was the Well Elderly study that demonstrated the value of an occupational approach, which included occupational therapy, to the lifestyle redesign for older people in America (Jackson, Carlson, Mandel, Zemke, & Clark, 1998). The results highlighted the benefits of engaging in personally meaningful occupations. This has been further supported by the Well Elderly 2 randomized controlled trial, which studied 460 older people in the United States aged 60 to 95 from ethnically diverse populations (Clark et al., 2011). This study provided evidence to support a 6-month preventative, lifestyle-oriented intervention by occupational therapists. It demonstrated a cost-effective approach that had a positive effect, particularly on mental well-being. It included weekly small-group sessions covering areas such as evaluating time use, rehearsal, transportation, social relationships, cultural awareness, and changing routines and habits. Developing such skills may not only promote mental well-being, but also may assist transition into retirement and contribute to maintaining a productive lifestyle.

Although occupational science maintains a relationship with occupational therapy, it has evolved and become a much more multidisciplinary discipline, with impact on academia, policy, and society in general. It is a discipline that is moving forward and generating knowledge and action regarding occupation that will have local and global implications (Laliberte Rudman et al., 2008).

Aging

There is no doubt that we are all living in an increasingly aging society. The World Health Organization (WHO) asserts that "the aging population is one of humanity's greatest triumphs" (2002, p. 6). Key facts suggested by the WHO (2012) indicate that the number of people today aged 60 and over has doubled since 1980. People aged 80 years will almost quadruple to 395 million between now and 2050. Within the next 5 years, adults aged 65 and over will outnumber children under the age of 5. By 2050, these older adults will outnumber all children under the age of 14. The majority of older people live in low- or middle-income countries, and by 2050, this number will have increased to 80%.

Older people can be valued and respected by those who know them well; however, attitudes to other older people within the broader community can be different (WHO, 2012). In traditional societies or settings, older people are more respected, and often viewed as elders. However, in some societies, older people are less revered, and are often marginalized. Societies that have enforced retirement ages may view older people as less energetic and less valuable to a potential employer (WHO, 2012).

Much of our thinking in Western society has focused on the burden of the aging population in terms of increased health and social care costs; however, there are alternatives to such views. Carlson et al. (1998, p. 108) found that existing research and our everyday observations indicated that an "outstanding" quality of life can be a realistic and achievable outcome for older people. Therefore, older people can be viewed as successfully aging, with a significant contribution to make to society and the workplace. Older people should be considered a valuable resource for their families, communities, and economies when they have access to supportive and enabling living environments (WHO, 2007).

By optimizing opportunities for health, participation, and security, we can enhance quality of life as people age (WHO, 2002). Research by Tatzer, Van Nes, and Jonsson (2012) indicates that older people do not always perceive themselves as old or sick, despite problems in mobility, the presence of chronic disease, and advanced age. This perception is associated with the person's engagement in occupation that is meaningful and linked to their identity. Engaging in occupation is the means to continue, test, and adapt to the aging self. Continued occupational engagement in relation to their own proximate world unconstrained by space and time is important in achieving occupational well-being for older people (Nilsson, Lundgren, & Liliequist, 2012). This world involves contact with family, friends, and society, as well as a shared norm to be independent.

WORK

Healthy living is said to involve blending work and pleasure (Holmes, 2007, p. 7). Work in itself is a multidimensional, complex phenomenon that has different representations and meanings dependent on culture, language, and circumstance. Some might say it is hard to define and agree on what actually constitutes *work* (O'Hallaran & Innes, 2005). Simply defined, it can be activity involving mental or physical effort done in order to achieve a result (Oxford dictionary online, n.d.). It can also mean paid employment, duties or tasks in a workplace, or productive activity (Holmes, 2007). For many, work is a major, sustainable component of life; it provides an income, promotes independence and security, and provides a structure to everyday life (Holmes, 2007). A work role can involve social contact and inclusion, enable people to make a valuable and worthwhile contribution to society and define a person in terms of status and self-identity (Holmes, 2007). An individual's motivation to work depends on relative extrinsic and intrinsic factors, the importance of which varies depending on the individual (O'Hallaran & Innes, 2005). Most people associate work with the extrinsic rewards of income and status. Csikszentmihalyi (1975) suggested that an intrinsically satisfying occupation induced a state of flow (i.e., a totally absorbing activity). Volti (2012) has offered the notion of occupational prestige, which is distinguished from status. *Prestige* in this context implies respect, admiration, and a hierarchical context. When we initially meet people, we often question them about their jobs, not only in an effort to start a conversation, but also to establish the contextual circumstances of the person. In the case of older people, we might pose the question, "What did you do when you were working?" This in itself may imply that the older person is no longer a productive member of society and could potentially have a detrimental effect. It may act as a reminder that the person no longer holds this role in society, and the status that it previously afforded him or her.

People working longer can be viewed as a solution to the maintenance of economic prosperity (Van Dalen, Henkens, & Schippers, 2010). For some, work may mean being in a job at a certain point in time, whereas for others, it may mean a long-term aspiration or career. For example, a student may work part-time as a waitress (job) in a café while working toward a graduate post in engineering (career).

Work does not always mean paid employment; volunteering has recognized benefits, not only for the volunteers, but for their families, service recipients, and the wider community (McNamara & Gonzales, 2011). Therefore, society and legislators need to recognize the possibilities and benefits of volunteer involvement (see Chapter 9). Work is one of the most effective means to improve the well-being of people, their families, and their communities, and it should be safe and accommodating (Waddell & Burton, 2006). Being without work can be destructive to self-respect, present risks for poor health (physical and mental), thwart the pursuit of happiness, and deplete well-being (Ansell, 2011). Occupational science recognizes this inextricable and fundamental link between health, well-being, occupation, and the development of occupations across the life span. We assume that work can be good for health, is socially desirable, and helps people to enjoy social engagement (Steward, 1996). Jakobsen describes getting older as a challenging occupational developmental stage when individuals can afford the "time and space to become more fully themselves, and to share with others the fruits and wisdom of their being" (2004, p. 125).

The current aging population is unprecedented, and without parallel in the history of humanity. Research published by the Organization for Economic Cooperation and Development (OECD, 2011) indicates that older workers are less likely to be employed than their prime-aged counterparts (age 25 to 50). The participation rates of older workers (age 50 to 64) in 31 countries averaged 63% in 2008, while rates of prime-aged workers averaged 75% in the same year. Participation rates for older workers exceed 70% in 7 countries, including Japan and the United States. However, Belgium, Hungary, Italy, Poland, and Turkey all have less than half of older workers active in the labor market.

Rates of older workers in most countries studied by the OECD were higher in 2008 than in 1970. In many cases, participation rates declined during the early part of the period from 1970 to 2008, a trend that was later reversed, typically in the last decade or so. Germany, Iceland, the Netherlands, and New Zealand saw the largest increases. In only 5 countries—France, Greece, Hungary, Poland, and Turkey—were participation rates lower in 2008 than they were in 1970.

It has been suggested that there is inconclusive empirical evidence regarding the relationship between age and productivity (Van Dalen, Henkens, & Schippers, 2010). Occupational science focuses on individual experiences and contextual dimensions—one of which is how life occupations change as people get older. Therefore, it may have some worth and provide new insights in terms of the study of work as a specific occupation (O'Hallaran & Innes, 2005).

WORK AND THE OLDER PERSON: AN OCCUPATIONAL PERSPECTIVE

Defining to a broad audience exactly what is meant by an *older worker* can be difficult. This is due to the differing working contexts, economic priorities, cultural significance, societal norms, state responsibilities, ages of retirement, and political drivers inherent in various nations. Riach (2011) has indicated that older workers may lose their employment opportunities due to their age, restructuring of organizations, downsizing of particular industries, and the longer-term unemployment of older people.

Older people also experience some challenges in relation to work. Barriers to work for the older person can include stress, over-reliance on qualifications, lack of employer support, physical demands of the workplace, difficulties gaining employment, and job security itself (Fraser, McKenna, Turpin, Allen, & Liddle, 2009). Occupational science can offer a further perspective, not only on the challenges, but also the consequences of not being able to engage in a productive lifestyle. The concepts of occupational science are discussed next, with illustrative narratives and case studies.

Occupational Deprivation

Occupational deprivation can be defined as the lack of occupational choices that is beyond the control of an individual (Wilcock, 1998) and occurs over an extended period of time (Whiteford, 1997). Older workers in Australia identified stress, lack of support, physical demands, and overemphasis on qualifications as barriers to their participation in work (Fraser et al., 2009), which lead to occupational deprivation.

Hocking (2012) refers to a study by Brown that describes a group of older women who are denied occupational opportunities, potentially resulting in occupational deprivation. These women followed their adult children to North America under reunification policies. Unable to access the social benefits of working, they presented with both psychological and physical health issues. Their younger families often expected that they would take on household and childcare roles, rather than education or paid employment opportunities. As a consequence, they had limited opportunities to develop their English language skills, and some reported being denied opportunities to attend English courses due to their age.

The brief story of Raj illustrates how occupational deprivation due to circumstances beyond a person's control can impact health, well-being, and employment opportunities:

> *Raj, aged 42, was a high school teacher is his native country. He was successful and well respected by his students and colleagues. His last post was as a deputy head teacher. His working environment was very supportive and affirming, and it gave him the recognition he deserved for his hard work and contributions to the education and management of others. The school and its community gave Raj and his family a social outlet, as well as a means of providing for the family financially.*
>
> *Due to family and political circumstances in his own country, it became necessary for Raj to relocate to the UK. He was unable to find a job as a teacher because his qualifications were not recognized or were not deemed suitable for any post in an education setting. Raj faced many barriers to gaining employment that had real meaning to him. He eventually took a low paid, unskilled job in a factory so that he could financially provide for his family. Raj felt lost and disempowered. The lack of recognition of his experience and education, in addition to a very unsupportive work environment, led to significant health problems related to his stress and depression. As a result, Raj had difficulty going to work on a full-time basis, which seriously impacted the family finances. Raj was occupationally deprived, with a consequential impact on his health and well-being.*

Occupational Alienation

Occupational alienation is a subjective experience where an individual may feel powerlessness, frustration, isolation, loss of control, and estranged from society (Wilcock, 1998). Research conducted in the Netherlands indicated that the productivity of older people was rated substantially lower than that of younger people in the workforce, with negative stereotypes toward older people being prevalent in the labor market (Van Dalen et al., 2010), thus potentially alienating a possible source of productive workers. Working Better, a study by the Equality and Human Rights Commission (2010) that was based on a telephone survey with 1500 people aged 50 to 75, found that half of older workers with poor health felt unable to approach their managers to discuss their situation. The consequence of this may be occupational alienation. Someone who loses his or her job may feel alienated from society, coworkers, friends, and work contacts. Change in role may also lead to occupational alienation, as is illustrated by Janet's story:

Janet had followed her husband around the world with his military career for many years. In each place she lived, she became involved in the community of Army wives, working on the bases while supporting her husband and living a fulfilling life. When her husband retired, they returned to live in the UK. Due to her life in the Army community, it was difficult for Jane to establish herself from an employment perspective; this made it hard for her to find a working role when her husband left the Army. She no longer had a ready-made community in which to maintain a productive role. In addition, her husband now wanted to take responsibility for the household, which was previously her domain. The consequence was a sense of loss and isolation, which led to alienation, and consequently depression.

It took some time for Janet to re-establish productive roles, which she accomplished through readjustment within her marriage and becoming an active member of a local volunteer organization. In her volunteer job, she provided support to a day care service for people with disabilities, regaining an occupational balance in her life.

Occupational Imbalance

Occupational imbalance refers to a loss of balance in those occupations that would normally be healthy for an individual. As Wilcock (1998) suggests, it is a loss of balance between physical, mental, and social occupations (chosen or obligatory), or between doing and being. Someone who is not working may spend more time in passive leisure pursuits, withdrawing, and doing very few productive activities. Alternatively, it is possible to overwork and have very little time for other occupations or roles.

When moving from paid employment to volunteer work or retirement, occupational imbalance may occur if the individuals do not feel able to say no to demands on their time. This is illustrated by Catherine, 66, a retired university lecturer:

I probably get tired a bit more quickly, but it's more that lots of things come together that I haven't really got any control over. If I'm doing something related to the university, it all seems to come at once. For example, last month I had external examining and a conference in Lithuania and…this is another thing—senior moments happen a lot more frequently— but there was another big thing as well. I would have preferred it to be spread around a bit more. November is nowhere near as bad.

Although this may be manageable in the short term, it can lead to health issues if it occurs over a prolonged period. Mike was also in danger of experiencing occupational imbalance when he returned to work on a temporary basis following retirement:

I retired at 60 from my main job as a shipping agent, but went back as a glorified office boy. The man who was doing it had to go into the hospital, so they asked me to go back for 3 or 4 months, but that became 2 years. I was opening the office up at 8 in the morning and leaving at 4:30 with a half hour for lunch. After 3 or 4 months, there was no sign of him coming back, so I said I would stay until Christmas. After that I said I would only do afternoons and they agreed, so I stayed for 2 years and that paid for my trip to Australia. In a way, I enjoyed it and I was helping them because when you work somewhere for 40 years you have a bit of loyalty to them. They wouldn't have got another silly bugger like me to do it!

Although Mike was assertive enough to ask for shorter work hours, for those who are not assertive, lack confidence, or are worried that they will be fired for making such a request, there is a danger that occupational imbalance with continue and lead to poor health.

Occupational Disruption

Occupational disruption is the inability to engage in occupations as a result of life events, acute illness, injury, or environmental changes (Whiteford, 1997). A person may have to temporarily stop working due to poor health or an injury at work, thus preventing his or her usual occupational roles and routines until the injury or illness is resolved. The experience Mike had before he retired is an example of occupational disruption:

> *I was happy in the job until I was about 56 or 57, and then we lost a lot of the services and the job wasn't the same. Because they all went to containers and the locks weren't wide enough to bring in the big containers, the work went elsewhere and I was just looking around for things to do.*

Recognizing the Potential of Older People at Work

There is transformation in current thinking in some countries recognizing the potential of older people to make valued contributions to work environment. Older people may be wiser and less impulsive and have better decision-making skills than their younger counterparts. Their ability to adapt and respond to both the possibilities and challenges in a working context should not be underestimated.

Occupational Adaptation

Crises may occur as people experience life events. Old age offers such potential crises that may disrupt lifelong occupational patterns (Odawara, 2010), leading people to negotiate and adapt to life events, or to be challenged and disadvantaged. There is no doubt that for most, the aging process can mean a decline in physical, sensory, and potentially cognitive capacity, and as a consequence, a decline in the ability to engage and participate in some occupations (see Chapters 4, 6, and 7). Older people must struggle against and adapt to such declines by using resources and strategies (Tatzer, Van Nes, & Jonsson, 2012). Overcoming difficulties such as physical decline can be done by exercising, for example. The adaptation of occupations can mean relinquishing previous occupations or finding alternative ways of performing them. Alternatively, an older person may discover new occupations or find new meaning in old occupations (Tatzer et al., 2012). Maintaining a healthy lifestyle, having a passion for work, and education are factors that support continued work (Fraser et al., 2009). Work is a legitimate opportunity for older people to remain economically active and socially included (Roberts, 2006), and the possibility for older people to adapt to the work environment should not be discounted. Alternatively, older individuals may want to adapt their employment to meet their needs. In a study by the Equality and Human Rights Commission (2010), 10% of men and 7% of women interviewed between the ages of 50 and 75 would like to set up their own businesses when they retire from mainstream employment. The study also highlighted that enthusiasm for learning persists, with one-third of participants aged 60 to 64 having undertaken training in the past 3 years, and 21% of persons over 50 having had training to improve their job prospects.

Occupational adaptation can be seen in the story of Rachel, 65, whose previous employment was as a lecturer in engineering. She has experienced long-term health problems affecting her mobility since her mid-20s.

> *Yes, things are taking more time, but how much is health and how much is advancing age, I don't know, and of course, medication keeps you going but it also had an impact, so it's balancing that. I think one key lesson is I'm not proud. It's ridiculous, some people say I wouldn't be seen dead with a stick or a scooter or a walker, but I've never bothered about that. Whatever adaptations I need, I've just had.*
>
> *I can manage myself with my adapted bathroom, hoist in the bedroom, etc. I have a power chair for the house when I'm tired, a scooter out there, and car for as long as I can drive it.*

> *So having those adaptations enables you to do your work role, as it conserves your energy?*
>
> *Absolutely it does and I find that liberating. It's just technology in another form and I'm happy with that, my life has been technology in one form or another. It's a servant, mobilizer, and enabler so why not?*

Occupational Potential

Wicks (2005) urges us to consider occupational potential following her life story research with 6 older women. She suggests that it is a highly complex construct—a multidimensional and dynamic human phenomenon that encompasses a person's needs and capacities. According to Wicks, occupational potential evolves over time, is unique to each person, and is influenced by both the person and his or her environment. This can involve an unpredictable trajectory due to both personal and environmental factors. She has proposed the following definition of occupational potential: "People's capacity to do what is required and what they have the opportunity to do, to become whom they have the potential to be" (p. 137). Therefore, older people should not be limited in terms of work opportunities, but encouraged to consider realistic possibilities in terms of their own capacity and contribution.

The story of Jim Clements, age 100, illustrates how being given an opportunity to return to work following retirement can help to sustain health and well-being. His occupational potential is clearly recognized by his colleagues and friends:

> *Jim Clements, who lives and works in Harlow, said he started the role at Active Security after his wife told him to get a job when he became bored following retirement. He said: "My wife got on me because I kept moaning and didn't know what to do with myself. I will hate it when I do pack up, but it's got to come one day."*
>
> *Mr. Clements, who turned 100 in January, spends 2 mornings a week at work. His roles include "filing, shredding, and making tea." He said, "I went for a month's trial and it progressed from there. I like everyone who works there, they are very, very good to me."*
>
> *Before he took retirement, Mr. Clements' jobs included making torpedoes. He became a widower 20 years ago and said the part-time job kept his mind active. His manager, Ray Le Monde, said he was an "absolutely excellent" member of staff and an "inspiration—he's a 100-year-old who still thinks he's 21." He said: "We have to rein him in sometimes and make him respect his age. He's very conscientious and willing to do more tasks than we will ever let him."*
>
> *Jackie Cowley also works at Active Security and says she is part of a group of friends who take turns looking after Mr. Clements. She said, "They won't let him finish work, they like to keep an eye on him to make sure he's all right. He has an active social life and a wicked sense of humor."* (BBC News Essex, 2013)

Occupational Enrichment

Occupational enrichment can be achieved by providing opportunities for people to engage in a range of occupations, either alone or within groups. This can include work that is paid or voluntary. It may also involve addressing wider, systemic organizational or institutional issues, such as policies on access to employment programs, and training and development (Cronin-Davis, Lang, & Molineux, 2003). Catherine (age 66) is involved in a range of occupations that include learning new skills and volunteering; this enriches her life.

> *My structured things now are, I volunteer on a chaplaincy team at the hospital on Wednesdays and Sundays, and I go to lip reading classes on Tuesday afternoon. This is my third year and I love it, they are a great group to work with. I have church-related activities*

at certain times during the week. Oh, and I head up the pastoral team in the church, so Monday is definitely for visiting some of the older folk in the church. But then someone will get admitted to the hospital....so there is plenty happening and I also have more time to meet with my friends.

Catherine also referred to the range of opportunities for continued work since retirement:

It keeps my brain active, I suppose. I don't read academic texts as much as I did, but that's because I don't write for journals like I did. I've been coauthor of an article in a supervisory role. Having said that, it's been 90 years since insulin was discovered and suddenly out of the blue my consultant has asked me to write a reflection on my experiences for a journal, so I've spent a little time reflecting on 56 years of having type 1 diabetes, which was absolutely priceless. I had to go back to find some quotes from the diabetic bible of 1956 and it was things like, "you can sharpen your needle on pummel stone and it will last you for a couple of months," so that was quite fascinating reading. I still get my professional journal, but it's been a while since I read one, so I don't have to do what I did before. But following this article, I now find that I'm presenting at a national diabetes conference in a couple of weeks on a similar sort of topic to 200 people, which will be nerve-wracking, and then next month I'm doing a spirituality and health talk at Durham. I'm afforded lots of opportunities from being known.

Occupational Justice

Occupational justice is based on the premise that all people should have access to the resources to engage in chosen or necessary occupations regardless of age, disability, gender, culture, or geographical location (Townsend & Wilcock, 2003). This equally applies to the working or social context. Older people do not stop contributing to their communities when they retire. In some areas, economic circumstances force older people to take paid work long after they should have left employment or retired (WHO, 2007). We should ensure an occupationally just society that affords older people work opportunities that are valued and contribute to the economic fabric of their communities. Older people should be recognized for the life and work experiences they can contribute to the workplace. There are many advantages to both the older person and the work community of continued employment, including income, social considerations, being occupied and having a purpose in a supportive workplace, emotional and physical well-being, using skills, and maintaining autonomy and independence (Fraser et al., 2009). This can be demonstrated again by Catherine, who has the opportunity for a small amount of paid work, and an extensive amount of voluntary work. Given that she has a high level of skill in her area, she perhaps has more opportunity for occupational justice than her contemporaries who are retiring from less skilled backgrounds.

I don't know if I actively planned to carry on working past retirement. I got my professorship a year before I finished, so from that point of view, I only had a year to work on that, but because I got that label I was able to be a research fellow and am now doing a PR job for the university. I don't get any funding for some of the conferences I go to, but I'm now a visiting professor at 2 European universities, so they pay my expenses to go there.

A further example is that of 98-year-old Dolly Saville, who has worked in the same pub for about 74 years, and is believed to be the world's oldest barmaid.

Dolly has worked at the Red Lion Hotel in Wendover, Buckinghamshire in the United Kingdom for about 74 years. She still works a lunch shift 3 days a week and says she "won't quit pulling pints until they throw me out." She became a great, great grandmother in November and said she would like to teach the baby the pub trade one day. Deputy manager Sam Hughes said: "Dolly is a real tourist attraction. We know she wants to work until she's at least 100, and we're certainly not going to ask her to leave." He described her as a "real asset" to the hotel. *"Dolly is as good as anyone else and likes to keep busy. She is just as important to the hotel today as she was 70 years ago." Dolly says, "There's no stopping, you just keep going. I love the work and I love the people here."*

Dolly, who will be 99 in April, started working at the Red Lion before World War II, but said she had not really wanted to work in a pub. "The boss asked me if I'd like a job and I said no, then he asked again and I said I'd give it a try."

Her daughter, Anne Edwards, 78, said her mother would like to teach great, great granddaughter Darcey Mae Dugan "how to pull a pint when she's old enough."

"There's a right way and a wrong way to pull a pint, and I can still do that properly at 98." She added, "I won't stop working unless they kick me out." (BBC News, 2013)

CONCLUSION

This chapter focused on how an occupational perspective might assist with appreciating the importance of work in this life stage. It has defined concepts related to occupational science and how this can be viewed in relation to the individual experience of work, and also their contribution to the workplace, economic fabric of society, and the community. Occupational science is a developing discipline that can offer useful insights into the work issues faced by older people. By recognizing and embracing the potential challenges that older people face and promoting a proactive approach, such challenges can be addressed and overcome.

REFERENCES

Ansell, M. (2011). A new dawn—new opportunities: Rethinking our attitudes to work and illness. *Health and Care Conference, Brighton.*

BBC News Essex. (2013, January 29). *100-year-old man continues to work after 'boring' retirement.* Retrieved April 8, 2013, from http://www.bbc.co.uk/news/uk-england-essex-21246855.

BBC News Beds, Herts & Bucks. (2013, January 25). *'Oldest' barmaid 'won't quit' Wendover pub job.* Retrieved April 8, 2013 from http://www.bbc.co.uk/news/uk-england-beds-bucks-herts-21200916.

Brown, C. A., (2008). The implications of occupational deprivation experienced by elderly female immigrants. *Diversity in Health and Social Care, 5,* 65-69.

Carlson, M., Clark, F., & Young, B. (1998). Practical contributions of occupational science to the art of successful aging: How to sculpt a meaningful life in older adulthood. *Journal of Occupational Science, 5*(3), 107-118.

Clark, F., Jackson, J., Carlson, M., Chou, C. P., Cherry, B. J., Jordan-Marsh, M., Azen, S. P. (2012). Effectiveness of a lifestyle intervention in promoting the well-being of independently living older people: Results of the Well Elderly 2 randomised controlled trial. *Journal of Epidemiology and Community Health, 66*(9), 782-790.

Cronin-Davis, J., Lang, M. & Molineux, M. (2003). Occupational science: the forensic challenge. In M. Molineux (Ed.), *Occupation for occupational therapists.* Oxford: Blackwell Publishing.

Csikszentmihalyi, M. (1975). *Beyond boredom and anxiety.* San Francisco: Jossey-Bass Publishers.

Equality and Human Rights Commission. (2010). *Working better: The over 50s, the new work generation.* Retrieved March 21, 2013, from http://www.equalityhumanrights.com/uploaded_files/publications/workingbetter_over_50s.pdf.

Fraser, L., McKenna, K., Turpin, M., Allen, S., & Liddle, J. (2009). Older workers: An exploration of the benefits, barriers and adaptations for older people in the workforce. *Work, 33*(3), 261-272.

Hocking, C. (2012). Working for citizenship: The dangers of occupational deprivation. *Work, 41*(4), 391-395.

Holmes, J. (2007). *Vocational rehabilitation.* Chichester, UK: Blackwell Publishing.

Jackson, J., Carlson, M., Mandel, D., Zemke, R., & Clark, F. (1998). Occupation in lifestyle redesign: The Well Elderly study occupational therapy program. *American Journal of Occupational Therapy, 52*(5), 326-336.

Jakobsen, K. (2004). If work doesn't work: How to enable occupational justice. *Journal of Occupational Science, 11*(3), 125-134.

Laliberte Rudman, D., Dennhardt, S., Fok D., Huot, S., Molke, D., Park, A., & Zur, B. (2008) A vision for occupational science: Reflecting on our disciplinary culture. *Journal of Occupational Science, 15*(3), 136-146.

McNamara, T. K., & Gonzales, E. (2011). Volunteer transitions among older adults: The role of human, social and cultural capital in later life. *The Journals of Gerontology Series B: Psychological Sciences and Social Sciences, 66*(4), 490-501.

Molineux, M. (2010). Occupational science and occupational therapy: Occupation at center stage. In C. Christiansen & E. Townsend (Eds.), *Introduction to occupation: The art and science of living* (2nd ed.). Upper Saddle River, NJ: Prentice Hall.

Nilsson, I., Lundgren, S., & Liliequist, M. (2012). Occupational well-being among the very old. *Journal of Occupational Science, 19*(2), 115-126.

Odawara, E. (2010). Occupations for resolving life crises in old age. *Journal of Occupational Science, 17*(1), 14-19.

OECD. (2011). "Trends in Retirement and in Working at Older Ages", In *Pensions at a Glance 2011: Retirement-income Systems in OECD and G20 Countries*. OECD Publishing. Retrieved March 22, 2013, from http://dx.doi.org/10.1787/pension_glance-2011-6-en.

O'Hallaran, D., & Innes, E. (2005). Understanding work in society. In C. Christiansen & E. Townsend (Eds.), *Introduction to occupation: The art and science of living*. Upper Saddle River, NJ: Prentice Hall.

Riach, K. (2011). Understanding the experience of the "older worker" in a globalized world. *Work, Employment & Society, 25*(4), 806-813.

Roberts, I. (2006). Taking age out of the work place: Putting older workers back in? *Work, Employment & Society, 20*(1), 67-86.

Shakespeare, W. (1623). Antony and cleopatra. Retrieved June 11, 2014, from http://shakespeare.mit.edu/cleopatra/full.html.

Steward, B. (1996). Unemployment and health 1: The impact of unemployment on clients in therapy and rehabilitation. *British Journal of Occupational Therapy, 3*(7), 360-363.

Tatzer, V., Van Nes, F., & Jonsson, H. (2012). Understanding the role of occupation in aging: Four life stories of older Viennese women. *Journal of Occupational Science, 19*(2), 138-149.

Townsend, E. (1997). *Enabling occupation: An occupational therapy perspective*. Ottawa, Canada: Canadian Association of Occupational Therapists.

Townsend, E., & Wilcock, A. (2003). Occupational justice. In C. Christiansen & E. Townsend (Eds.), *Introduction to occupation: The art and science of living*. Upper Saddle River, NJ: Prentice Hall.

Van Dalen, H., Henkens, K., & Schippers, J. (2010). Productivity of older workers: Perceptions of employers and employees. *Population and Development Review, 36*(2), 309-330.

Volti, R. (2012). *An introduction to the sociology of work and occupations* (2nd ed.). London: Sage Publications.

Waddell, G., & Burton, K. (2006). *Is work good for your health and well-being?* London: The Stationery Office.

Whiteford, G. (1997). Occupational deprivation and incarceration. *Journal of Occupational Science, 4*(3), 126-130.

Wicks, Q. A. (2005). Understanding occupational potential. *Journal of Occupational Science, 12*(3), 130-139.

Wilcock, A. (1998). *An occupational perspective of health*. Thorofare, NJ: SLACK Incorporated.

Work [def. 1]. (n.d.). In *Oxford dictionaries online*. Retrieved January 3, 2013, from http://oxforddictionaries.com/definition/english/work.

World Health Organization. (2002). *Active ageing: A policy framework*. Retrieved February 16, 2013, from http://whqlibdoc.who.int/hq/2002/WHO_NMH_NPH_02.8.pdf.

World Health Organization. (2007). Global age-friendly cities: A guide. Retrieved January 2, 2013, from http://www.who.int/aging/publications/Global_age_friendly_cities_Guide_English.pdf.

World Health Organization. (2012). *Knowledge Translation Framework for Ageing and Health*. Retrieved April 8, 2013, from http://www.who.int/aging/publications/knowledge_translation.pdf.

Yerxa, E., Clark, F., Jackson, J., Parham, D., Pierce, D., Stein, C., & Zemke, R. (1989). An introduction to occupational science: A foundation for occupational therapy in the 21st century. *Occupational Therapy in Health Care, 6*(4), 1-17.

Theories of Aging

Linda A. Hunt, PhD, OTR/L, FAOTA

The more I want to get something done, the less I call it work.—Richard Bach (1977)

With the explosion of interprofessional research on aging comes more new theories of aging. Numerous aging theories have been developed to explain what is observed in various disciplines, including biology, anthropology, gerontology, psychology, sociology, and social work. Theorizing is a process of developing ideas that allow understanding and explanation of empirical observations. Bengtson, Gans, Putney, and Silverstein (2009) refer to theories as lenses. These lenses can provide numerous ways of interpreting observations. This chapter will explore some well-developed theories of aging, how they apply to older people working past retirement age, and propose a new theory. This new theory is based not on a linear life span consisting of distinct years for education, work, family, and leisure, but rather a life plan in which education, work, family, and leisure exist in different proportions throughout life. The theory is based on the assumption that the Baby Boomers will engage in different life pursuits that bring purpose to their lives at different times throughout their lives. This proposed theory is called the "Purposeful Theory of Aging," and was developed through the lens of this author, an occupational therapist. Its premise supports the idea that employment and volunteering contribute to an individual's identity through intrinsic and social beliefs of usefulness, which give life meaning.

Retirement is defined as withdrawal from one's position or occupation or from active working life, and the exit from an organizational position or career path of considerable duration (Merriam-Webster's online dictionary, n.d.). Motivation to continue working after retirement may be due to intrinsic values or financial concerns. An intrinsic value may surround the strong need to be useful to others, an observation not fully explored in theories of aging. This chapter discusses 5 theories of aging in the context of employment past retirement age, including Identity Theory Continuity Theory of Aging, Activity Theory of Aging, and Disengagement Theory of Aging, plus my proposed theory, Purposeful Aging Theory. This last theory centers around the question, "How useful have I been?" The theory is tied into the practice and research on reminiscence (Parker,

Hunt LA, Wolverson C.
Work and the Older Person: Increasing Longevity and Well-Being (pp 25-36).
© 2015 SLACK Incorporated.

1995; Webster, Bohlmeijer, & Westerhof, 2010). One of the important questions in reviewing one's life is to answer this question to oneself and possibly to others. To better understand this proposed theory, let us look at aging theories that attempt to explain the thought processes and behaviors of aging persons as applied to aging workers.

IDENTITY THEORY

Tajfel (1978) notes that Identity Theory has gained popularity in the organizational sciences. Much focus has been on role identity as it refers to "components of the self that correspond to the social roles we play" (Grube & Piliavin, 2000, p. 1109). For example, in the work environment, a member of a work team may identify herself as the implementer of the team. She is the one who puts ideas into action and prides herself on this role identity. Other team members look to her to get ideas activated, and she derives self-esteem from this role and ability. This may contribute to other role identities that stem from this primary role, such as organizer and leader.

Stryker and Statham (1985) have proposed a description of Identity Theory that postulates that within physical and social environments, people classify themselves and others according to their social roles. Every person occupies multiple roles, which are arranged in order of importance, and are associated with behavioral expectations unique to the dimensions of that role. Role identity is closely allied to perceptions of self, and thus people may seek legitimization of roles to which they are committed (Siebert, Mutran, & Reitzes 1999). Consequently, roles and their importance are stable across time and situations (Stryker & Burke, 2000), and people will seek situations in which their role perceptions are reinforced. Stryker and Burke (2000) argue that the Identity Theory must include both social structural and internal self-processes. Each influences the process of self-verification. Many of our roles affect the relationship between self and society, and how we verify our own view of ourselves. For example, our roles could be as parent, spouse, friend, coworker, owner, or supervisor. The list of all of our roles is endless and each may bring meaning and self-identity. Unfortunately, as one ages, one may begin to lose some roles. For example, through divorce or death, one may no longer be a spouse. As friends and neighbors move or die, or children become adults, one further loses more valuable social roles.

Through working, one may continue life roles, including valued social roles and intrinsic roles of feeling useful that contribute to identity. For example, at work one interacts with coworkers or clients, which continues to socially engage the employed. When meeting new people this question often comes up: "What do you do?" This frequently asked question might project the belief that our activities, especially employment, contribute to role identity. Ann's story illustrates this theory:

> *Beginning in childhood, Ann thought about work and careers. She wanted to become a teacher. Daydreaming led her to think about becoming a university professor after an older cousin came to visit and talked about her experiences at a university. She visited the local university campus and saw herself walking across campus as a student and then as a professor. After achieving these lifelong goals, Ann moved from a large metropolitan city in the midwest to a small resort town in the northwest part of the United States. While living in the midwest, she had engaged in a vibrant career as an associate professor and director of a program at a university. She earned her PhD at the age of 50, and was excited about that accomplishment. Her days were filled with teaching, mentoring, solving problems, research and writing, and service. At age 51, a lifelong desire to live in a smaller community led to the decision to move. It was to be a new adventure. Ann was not thinking of her roles or identity; she was thinking of living in a beautiful place, making a change, and new opportunities. When meeting new people in this new community, the usual question arose: "What do you do?" She explained that she had a PhD and that she was a professor and director at a university in the midwest. This was the identity that she still carried with her. Upon hearing*

this, a woman replied, "No one here cares about that." Ann reported that she was speechless in response. This woman just stated that Ann's identity no longer mattered. Ann confided that she instantly felt worthless after years of working hard and earning her PhD fairly late in life. She reported, "I still see myself as a professor, a role that provided opportunities to impact lives through my teaching abilities. Furthermore, as the director of a program, I graduated students who were able to secure employment in a field that provided essential health care. I was known for my research, which contributed to the well-being of others."

Stower, Pervewe, and Munyon (2011) report that if an identity takes 100% psychological occupancy, then threats to that identity will likely have detrimental psychological effects. Conversely, if an identity takes only 10% of psychological occupancy, then a threat to that identity will likely have little detrimental psychological effect. At age 60, Ann explained that this comment was the former, a 100% threat to her identity. She went on to report:

I needed to do something before negative psychological effects set in. With this challenge to my identity from this woman, I went on a path to regain it. I soon became employed at a community college, returning to my previous role identity, my purpose, and what I believed was my usefulness to others. From there, I became a professor at another university and a director of a program. I was back 100%, and my role identity was no longer threatened. I have continued this role for the last 11 years. Now, I am 62 years old and I cannot imagine retiring fully. This is who I am.

The Identity Theory links to the Continuity Theory of Aging because individuals begin in childhood to seek future identities through career choices. Furthermore, people continue with those activities that give meaning, at which they excel, and that contribute to their self-identity. People will seek situations and activities in which their role perceptions are reinforced. As the case study above shows, this was true for Ann.

CONTINUITY THEORY OF AGING

The principle of continuity suggests that what people have done in the past indicates with high probability what they will do in the future. The Continuity Theory of Aging proposes that people who age most successfully are those who carry forward the habits, preferences, lifestyles, activities, and relationships from midlife into late life. The theory proposes that variables measured in midlife are strong predictors of outcomes in later life, and that many psychological and social characteristics are stable across the life span. Robert Atchley, the developer of this theory, writes:

Continuity Theory holds that, in making adaptive choices, middle-aged and older adults attempt to preserve and maintain existing internal and external structures; and they prefer to accomplish this objective by using strategies tied to their past experiences of themselves and their social world. Change is linked to the person's perceived past, producing continuity in inner psychological characteristics as well as in social behavior and in social circumstances. Continuity is thus a grand adaptive strategy that is promoted by both individual preference and social approval. (Atchley, 1989, p. 183)

The caveat to this is that these habits, preferences, lifestyles, activities, and relationships that are carried throughout life must be healthy choices. Carrying over poor health choices or having a job that contributes to poor health will not contribute to longevity.

Bridge employment defines the transition into part-time, self-employment, or temporary work after full-time employment ends and permanent retirement begins (Shultz, 2003). Von Bonsdorff, Shultz, and Leskinen (2009) link bridge employment to the Continuity Theory of Aging. The theory suggests that individuals who have been deeply involved in their work will try to sustain their daily routines by participating in activities that they value highly. Moreover, individuals who have been highly committed to their jobs are more likely to seek continuity through some form of participation in work life (Atchley, 1989). The work environment offers a natural way to maintain daily routines and engage in social interaction with colleagues, supervisors, and clients. For some individuals, maintaining these networks can influence the decision to continue at work instead of retiring early. Bridge employment might offer an opportunity to keep up these social contacts and networks after full-time employment ends.

Mr. Fine provides an example of the Continuity Theory of Aging with ties to the Identity Theory of Aging, as reported by his daughter:

> *His continued activities and occupations were selling and merchandising. While serving in the Army during WWII, Mr. Fine supervised 17 men who worked in the canteen selling items to the soldiers. After the war, as a salesman, phone calls were a major part of Mr. Fine's job. He notified clients of payments due from purchases, handled new sales at the small department store, and even scheduled times when he could go to the client's home and pick up a payment. These calls were made in the evening. A family member reported that there was great enthusiasm in his voice while he talked on the telephone to clients; Mr. Fine liked to socialize and he liked to talk. He retired at age 65 due to health issues. Because he viewed himself as a salesperson (Identity Role Theory), the lifelong activities he chose to continue were talking on the phone and selling. He secured a part-time job in phone sales, therefore bridging his retirement. When driving himself to work was no longer an option, he adapted the employment to his needs by having the owner of the company pick him up. Later, in his 70s, he stayed home and sold services and scheduled appointments for a pesticide company over the telephone. Hence, the job was adapted further for his increased age and health issues. Mr. Fine continued what he loved to do: selling and talking to people. He adapted his occupation by arranging transportation when he could no longer drive himself to work. Later, he stayed home and used technology to connect with customers. The enthusiasm and energy in his voice remained.*

As the above example shows, continuity helps as an adaptive strategy for dealing with age-related changes. To the extent that change builds upon, and has links to, the person's past, change is a part of continuity. Continuity is not the opposite of change. Rather, change and adaptation may exist with a connection to the individual's past. A strategy of successful aging may be maintaining activities and attitudes of middle age as long as possible by finding ways to adapt and continue the activities and roles. However, sometimes successful aging relies on substitutes for work when work is no longer an option. For example, a substitution that includes past activities, skills, and roles might include volunteer work (see Chapter 8). The next theory, Activity Theory of Aging, offers retirement as a way to provide opportunity to explore a new career that may not consist or rely on previous skills. The theory proposes new potential in old age to learn and participate in new activities that may contribute to cognitive and physical well-being.

ACTIVITY THEORY OF AGING

Havighurst (1961) proposed that people age most successfully when they participate in a variety of activities. This theory may explain the surge of volunteerism and senior activism in the 1960s and 1970s. It may also have been partly responsible for public policies, which underwrote the development of senior centers and other recreational facilities in that period. Successful aging may equal active aging. Activity engagement may be physical or intellectual in nature. The theory indicates that to maintain a positive self-image, the older person must develop new interests, hobbies, roles, and relationships to replace those that are diminished or lost in late life.

As roles change, the individual finds substitute activities for those roles. The Activity Theory readily fits into the life stage of retirement, as older people embrace new ways of living and engagement in life. In addition, it fits into the desire to continue employment by embracing new activities within work environments. However, this theory does not capture the entire picture of older people. It does not address the aging process and the fact that some older people may not have the physical or mental capacity to embrace new activities in the work environment. For example, getting to work may be challenging due to the inability to drive or use public transportation. Finally, for some, embracing new work activities that take them away from their habits and routines at work may be too stressful. An example is using new technology to do a routine task that one has done for over 30 years.

Activity Theory suggests that activity is preferable to inactivity because it facilitates well-being on multiple levels. With improved general health and prosperity in the older population, remaining active is more feasible now than when this theory was first proposed by Havighurst nearly 6 decades ago. The Activity Theory is applicable for a stable, postindustrial society that offers its older members many opportunities for meaningful participation in the work environment. However, it does not provide a complete theory for healthy aging. It seems to miss underlying infrastructure (i.e., transportation, availability of desired activities, and opportunities at work to assume new activities) for how older adults are enabled to participate in a variety of activities.

DISENGAGEMENT THEORY OF AGING

Disengagement Theory of Aging is based on the observation that as people grow older, they generally curtail their involvement in the activities of middle age. Cummings and Henry (1961) suggested in the Disengagement Theory that aging is an inevitable, mutual withdrawal or disengagement, resulting in decreased interaction between the aging person and others. This theory has historical significance in the study of aging, as it was the first theory developed to examine the behaviors of older people. Bonder (2009) points out that the theory was based on research with recent retirees, who would be expected to report disengaging from activity because they had just retired and became removed from activities that provided identity.

The story of Mrs. Cole demonstrates withdrawal from social involvement with others, due to having restricted opportunities to interact with other people after retirement. For some, work provides opportunities for socialization, and this socialization may be the only regular interaction that an employee finds.

> *Mrs. Cole worked as a receptionist and administrative assistant for an insurance company. She began working at this company when she was 40 years old, after her divorce. She retired at age 65, just because she thought that it was expected of her. For over 25 years, she had attended annual company picnics, bringing her children until they outgrew the desire to go, and attended the weddings, funerals, and birthday parties of coworkers. In addition, she often went out to dinner with several female coworkers. Her two grown children had moved to other parts of the country due to work or family demands. When she first retired, she continued to meet with her former coworkers for dinners out. After a year, one of them quit working for the company to be a caregiver to her husband, and another quit because her husband retired and they wanted to move closer to their grown children. She found that she had less and less in common with the few women that remained in the social group. She could no longer really talk about work, and they did not seem interested in what she did on a daily basis.*
>
> *Mrs. Cole had never reached out to strangers for friendships. When she married, she took on her husband's friends. Later, she made friends with the parents of her children's friends. These relationships discontinued over time as situations changed. Her coworkers were her natural friends. Her limited social interactions due to retirement resulted in disengagement. She found herself becoming lonely and watching too much television. She put on weight, and*

there were days that she did not leave the house. She traveled to visit her family; however, these visits were temporary, and at times she felt like an outsider. She also felt that her visits changed their routines, and this caused conflicts at times. Mrs. Cole thought about returning to work. Her daughter suggested enrolling in computer courses at the community college near her home. Going to classes provided her with a routine. She was hopeful that she would find volunteer work or paid employment where she was around people again.

Sometimes, retirement provides more time to participate in negative behaviors, and disengagement occurs, as Mr. Adler's story illustrates.

Mr. Adler worked at a manufacturing plant for 40 years. At age 63, he had a minor stroke and retired, collecting his pension and Social Security. Before retirement, his routine was to meet his work buddies at a tavern down the street from the manufacturing plant. Because his shift ended at 3:30 pm, he usually stayed at the tavern till 5:00 pm. He would then go home and have dinner with his family. For the last 15 years, it was just his wife and himself. Now that he was no longer working, he started drinking at home. He would drink a six-pack of beer every day before his wife arrived home from her job. This contributed to more health issues, and he became argumentative with everyone, including his wife. His wife no longer wanted to socialize with others because he would embarrass her with his negative behaviors. She had hoped to retire at age 65, but now wondered about the life she would have if she stayed home with her husband.

In her book, *Number Our Days,* Barbara Myerhoff (1978) discusses how people come to life when someone looks at them. She goes on to say that the people she wrote about "sought to establish their relative worth" (Myerhoff, 1978, p. 143). People crave an audience to witness their lives. Rather than disengaging in later years, they want people to know that their lives had meaning. Perhaps older people do not disengage themselves as the theory states, but rather, people disengage from them. We see this in nursing homes, where residents try to get attention, if only for someone to look at them. The Purposeful Aging Theory focuses on the importance of doing and being involved, and that most people crave a witness to all they have accomplished.

PURPOSEFUL AGING THEORY

It usually begins in early adolescence and continues throughout the life span: questioning the purpose of life. We ask, "Why am I here? What is my purpose?" Many books have been written to help us answer these questions. One book that comes to mind is *Man's Search for Meaning* by Viktor Frankl, which was first published in 1946 in Austria. Frankl believed that man's deepest desire is to search for meaning and purpose. Frankl wrote, "Everyone has his own specific vocation or mission in life to carry out, a concrete assignment which demands fulfillment. Therein he cannot be replaced, nor can his life be repeated. Thus, everyone's task is as unique as is his specific opportunity to implement it" (1984, p. 131). He also wrote that being jobless is being useless, and therefore lacking meaning in life. While in a concentration camp, he attributed his survival to finding meaning in the work that he was made to do. Later in life, as a medical doctor, he treated depression by having his patients engage in work or volunteer activities. Frankl believed in the need to teach these messages to future generations through writing and publishing. This desire to teach the next generation has been developed into a theory of personality development that resonates with the Purposeful Aging Theory.

Erik Erikson also wrote about the desire to teach the next generation, and introduced the concept of generativity in the context of a life span theory of personality development. According to Erikson, *generativity* "is primarily the concern in establishing and guiding the next generation" (1963, p. 267). Humans need to be productive and maintain meaning throughout the life span. Connectedness to future generations and to one's own life's meaning throughout the life span increases the salience of the identity (Identity Theory). It links lives to events, accomplishments, and people (Continuity Theory). Connectedness brings new activities into people's lives as they strive to learn new skills and ideas, and meet new people (Activity Theory). Finally, it delays or prevents disengagement in life (Disengagement Theory), as people may have a fundamental need for contact with others, and the goal of continuing to perform useful deeds. By being productive and engaged, people develop and maintain interactions and relationships with others, forming a network, even if it is only with a few people that provide support. This brings meaning to our lives, and ultimately enables survival. The horror of being frail and old is isolation. When older people no longer are able to contribute, and family and friends are distant or no longer living, life seems to be over.

There is a wonderful case report that illustrates this in *Number Our Days*. Myerhoff records a story of the importance of work in the chapter about Shmuel the tailor, who wants to tell his story for future generations. He wants future generations to understand what being the best at one's job really means. Wanting to be the best at his job as a tailor, he reports: "A coat is not an ordinary garment. It was our people who brought coats to the world. Before the little Jewish tailors came to America, what poor person could have a coat?" (p. 43). Myerhoff comments: "Creativity and seriousness belonged to work. It was both religion and play. When he worked, his imagination was freed" (p. 43). Shmuel goes on to say:

> The man who doesn't like his work is a slave, a slave to boredom. Maybe for him, retirement is a different kind of life. But in my life, I have never been bored. If you cannot tell a story to yourself when you are sewing, you are lost anyway. The work has no beginning and no end, but the story is told, it goes on in the head. A needle goes in and out. You hold a thread in your fingers. It goes to the garment, to the fingers, to the one who wears the garment, all connected. This is what matters, not whether you are paid for what you do. (p. 47)

One should do work with attention, care, and imagination—universal values. Myerhoff (1978) goes on to say:

> ...your description of the attitude you bring to your work will have meaning for many people. It's a valuable lesson for anyone. No matter what one's task, it can be done as described, so that finally peeling potatoes, any routine job, instead of being monotonous, becomes full of possibilities. (p. 66)

After telling his stories about work and growing up in a Polish village, Shmuel died knowing that his stories were recorded for others. Shmuel's narrative is a message that younger generations need to hear about work: No matter what one's job, it needs care and attention, because the end product or service goes to another person. It may be through one's work ethic that one contributes to and assumes responsibility for the next generation. McAdams and de St. Aubin (1992) wrote that the creation of a self-defining legacy that may be offered to society and to succeeding generations comes in part through one's work and employment. Often, in the work environment, there is a desire to nurture, assist, or be of some use to other people. Stewart, Franz, and Layton (1988) identified productivity as one of four main themes in generative content, and McAdams (1985) emphasized that generativity, unlike simple altruism or general prosocial behavior, involves the creation of a product or legacy. To measure generativity, McAdams and de St. Aubin (1992) developed the Loyola Generativity Scale. The Purposeful Aging Theory builds on their groundwork.

Helping people to find employment, and hence begin their legacy, may be an example of a perfect job. This is illustrated by Bess Fine, who, when asked what she liked best about her job, responded:

> "What did I like best about my job? I changed people's lives for the better. For example, I called on an employer to get a job order. The employer managed a beauty supply shop. She had a daughter who was 17 and had a baby. The daughter was working at a fast food restaurant. Her mother explained that the daughter always liked to work with tools, not girl's things. So I went to McDonnell Douglas and told Mrs. Golden, who worked in the HR

dept, about this girl who loved to work with tools and mechanical things. Mrs. Golden called her for an interview and she saw to it that this girl got her GED. Then they hired her and paid for her to go to college. She became a mechanical engineer at McDonnell Douglas, and met and married another engineer there. One of my happy endings." Mrs. Fine went on to explain that she had to work due to financial need. She believed that women who volunteered received all the "accolades for doing good deeds." She expressed this more than once: "I couldn't do volunteer work because my family needed my income from work. However, I believe I helped people and did just as much good as those who volunteer and do not receive pay. I am happiest when I am contributing. I contributed to the public's welfare and to the welfare of my family."

Mrs. Fine worked until she was 70 years old. She retired due to lung cancer, which she conquered. However, she decided that because she had been gone from work for several months, she would formally retire. She certainly contributed to the well-being of future generations through her work. She became employed due to financial necessity at age 40, but it was not the first time she was employed. She always sought employment to support herself and her family. Now, with this last job, she found her legacy—helping others find work. The desire to continue working past traditional retirement age provided continued purpose and financial security as she moved through her older years. All the way to age 93, she continued matching skills and personalities to specific jobs for family and friends. Frail and unable to physically leave her apartment for long periods of time, the telephone became her vehicle to maintain purpose as she gave advice over the phone. She took better care of herself to maintain her ability to contribute. This underscores the importance of the Purposeful Aging Theory, as it postulates that health may correlate to the current contributions to others through one's employment. This case study is an example that supports the research findings of Gruenewald, Liao, and Seeman (2012). Feeling needed and having socially valued skills in old age may contribute to longevity.

Another example is that of David Feffer, who retired at age 61, but did not stay in retirement long. As an entrepreneur, he started another business; however, this time the business was a nonprofit. As the owner of a startup nonprofit, Feffer does not receive pay, yet he puts as much time and passion into this new foundation as he did in his previous work. There is a trend for people who have been entrepreneurs all their lives to continue this desire to build something new after retirement. Feffer's startup, Crown of the Continent Guitar Foundation, is an organization that promotes the art and teaching of guitar music. It is still in its infancy, but growing each year.

At age 64, Mr. Feffer illustrates several positive aging theories. First, wanting to help others, being creative, working collaboratively, and starting something new links him to the Continuity Theory. Second, he has a strong identity as a vital, energetic contributor, which ties him to the Identity Theory because he wants to maintain how he thinks of himself as he ages. Third, his enjoyment of new learning leads Mr. Feffer to embrace new activities and meet new people, illustrating the Activity Theory of Aging. Most likely, no disengagement will occur in his life span. Finally, Feffer is driven by purpose, exemplifying the Purposeful Theory of Aging. The following is the narrative from his interview.

> **Please provide a short description of your current employment.**
> *Officially retired—cofounder and Chairman of Crown of the Continent Guitar Foundation; senior advisor to Array Health, a Seattle-based health care software company; advisor to Zinc Air, a Montana-based energy storage company; Vice chair of North Valley Hospital; board member of Bigfork Center for the Performing Arts. No salary is received from any of these.*

> **What are your earliest memories about working? What do you remember about people in your family working?**
> *My earliest memories about working are having regular chores at home in return for weekly allowance, shoveling snow for homes in our neighborhood, and carrying groceries*

to people's cars and homes for tips. All are positive memories—I enjoyed offering a service and being paid for a job well done. I also helped lead an annual neighborhood fair for different charities each year. My father was a surgeon and was on call 24/7. He loved what he was doing and was highly regarded by patients and colleagues. My mother volunteered in the Washington, D.C. community and at our school—she had a passion for service to the community.

What was your first job? How did you get the job? What did you learn from this first job in the way of skills? What did you learn from this job about future employment?

My first real job was at 16 working as the orderly for the Urology Department at George Washington University Hospital for the summer. I had been set for another job in the mail room at the White House but it fell through at the last minute. My father was a surgeon at GW, put the word out that I needed a job, and the Urology Department was looking for someone. I learned about understanding and helping meet people's needs through interaction with patients and staff; that any job, no matter how menial or unpleasant, was important; and professionalism and expertise through working with highly professional nurses and world-class surgeons. I learned that I enjoyed and was good at working with people and wanted to help make a difference in people's lives.

Tell me how education played a role in your ideas about employment while growing up.

I am not sure that my education played a direct role in my ideas about employment. Through my education, however, I became aware that I thrived on finding the answers to unanswered questions, like challenging the status quo, that I got bored if not challenged, that I learned in an atypical manner, and that I liked group projects.

What was your favorite job and why?

My favorite job was starting and running my own private company. I enjoyed coming up with an idea to address a significant societal need and inventing a new industry to meet that need, and creating an organization and work environment where everyone worked in a collaborative effort and could thrive and achieve their potential. I was doing what I wanted to do with people I liked, and I enjoyed it a great deal.

What motivates you to keep working beyond retirement age?

I don't think about what I do as work. I do what I do because I enjoy creating things, working with people, making a positive difference in my community, and learning.

How does this continued work affect your quality of life?

It energizes me, connects my wife and me to new and interesting people, continually gives me things to look forward to, and helps keep me "young," particularly when I'm working with good, smart people in their 20s, 30s, and 40s.

How does this continued work affect your image of yourself?

In two ways that are at the opposite end of the spectrum: I think of myself as young and vital. At the same time, I find that I have gotten to a point of experience and knowledge where I am offering wisdom that is viewed as valuable to people who are at an earlier stage in their careers.

Are you giving up anything that you value to continue to work?

At times yes, such as hiking, my guitar playing, and relaxed time with family. My family pushed me last year to slow down a bit. However, I do not give up the really important things, and I work to maintain balance. There was a situation last year where my wife and I wanted to visit our grandson. I had not seen him for a while. I considered not going because of Guitar Foundation activities, but very quickly concluded that time with our grandson came first. I am restructuring my commitments and roles to achieve better balance.

What in your past are you carrying over into your new role, as far as identities or continued activities?

I am carrying over my 40 years of health care experience in working with the Seattle health care software company and serving on the North Valley Hospital Board. I am carrying over my life long interest in music and entrepreneurial skills with the Guitar Foundation. And I am carrying on my life long charitable and community interests in a variety of ways in our home community.

What is new and different that you are embracing in this new role?

I knew absolutely nothing about the music industry, nor did I have any contacts or relationships. I had to jump in and learn from scratch. In many of my roles, I am an advisor/ consultant rather than having operational responsibility.

Describe how this new role might provide you with personal purpose.

Probably the two points are continually learning and looking forward to something, and making a difference in my community.

What would you say continued employment provides the most for you: reaffirms your identity? Provides continuity in your life? Keeps you engaged in activities? Provides purpose to your life?

In addition to the two things listed, work provides my wife and me with a connection to interesting people with whom we enjoy spending time, and to our community, and also provides an opportunity to make a positive difference.

CONCLUSION

Theories about aging and longevity are conceptualized as reflecting genetic, behavioral, and environmental effects. Analyzing these influences can be challenging, particularly when taking a life span perspective. This chapter introduced key behavioral theories of aging and applied them to engagement in employment. The Identity Theory (Stryker & Statham, 1985) may view the occupational role as a major source of personal validation, and the loss of the work role may be a wrenching experience that deprives the individual of a job, status, and a meaningful role in society. The Activity Theory (Havinghurst & Albrecht, 1953) stresses a continued dynamic involvement in the events of the individual's world. When roles and activities are relinquished, new useful roles and activities must take their place. The Continuity Theory (Atchley, 1989) explores the process of becoming an adult—the individual habits, preferences, commitments, and associations that are developed, and other dispositions that become a part of one's personality. As one grows older, there is a predisposition toward maintaining continuity in ways and commitments that are familiar to the individual. Work feeds our rituals (those procedures that are followed consistently), our habits (those activities that occur automatically and subconsciously), and finally our routines (what is done on a regular basis).

Continuity must be achieved throughout life. Experiences, traditions, and interests keep resurfacing from childhood throughout life. Work may play a part in allowing a person to remain the same person throughout his or her life. Mutual withdrawal from society and other people describes the Disengagement Theory (Cummings & Henry, 1961). The number of interrelationships between a person and other members of society are reduced, and those remaining are altered in quality. Again, when employment stops, it may be that society disengages from the retired person, when that person does not or cannot seek out new experiences. Older people need to be with others for successful aging (Rowe & Kahn, 1997).

This chapter has proposed a conceptual theory of aging called the Purposeful Aging Theory. This theory considers the way people need to be seen, and the ways in which the retirement culture offers and withholds that visibility. This proposed theory focuses on bringing purpose to our lives through work, and educating future generations on how we can give meaning to employment, which may then provide an identifiable purpose to our lives. Vaillant points out (in Trafford, 2004), "a career is not just a job but your defining purpose, the core of your being" (p. 14). He said employment could be a combination of work and family, the place where you find contentment, compensation, competence, and commitment. The Purposeful Aging Theory may encompass other theories of aging, as purpose may include self-identity, the roles we want to fulfill such as being a provider for oneself and family members; our activity engagement, as this helps structure our habits, routines, social interactions, and desires, giving meaning to everyday task; and our continued connection to society, believing we are contributing beyond our contributions to family and friends.

Through exploration of this theory, it may be found that the current older cohort of women may be able to maintain more continuity in their lives than men, who may be pulled away from the public world of work due to an accepted retirement age culture. Research will have to further develop this hypothesis and theory on how purposeful working into old age promotes successful aging. It will require interdisciplinary research and reflection, drawing on perspectives from occupational therapy, sociology, psychology, epidemiology, and other fields to consider how participation in work may be a factor that is associated with successful aging. It may lead to evidence-based interventions that help solve aging-related problems concerning employment engagement in old age.

REFERENCES

Atchley, R. C. (1989). A continuity theory of normal aging. *The Gerontologist, 29*(2), 183-190.

Bach, R. (1977). *Illusions: The Adventures of a Reluctant Messiah.* Newburyport: Hampton Roads.

Bengtson, L., Gans, D., Putney, N. M., & Silverstein, M. (2009). *Handbook of theories of aging* (2nd ed). New York: Springer.

Bonder, B. R. (2009). Meaning occupation in later life. In B. R. Bonder & V. Dal Bello-Haas (Eds.), *Functional performance in older adults* (pp. 45-62). Philadelphia: F.A. Davis Company.

Cummings, E. M., & Henry, W. E. (1961). *Growing old: The process of disengagement.* New York: Basic Books.

Erikson, E. H. (1963). *Childhood and society* (2nd ed.). New York: Norton.

Frankl, V. (1984). *Man's Search for Meaning* (p. 131). New York: Simon and Shuster Press.

Gruenewald, T. L., Liao, D. H., & Seeman, T. E. (2012). Contributing to others, contributing to oneself: Perceptions of generativity and health in later life. *Gerontology B Psychology Science Social Science. 67*(6), 660-665.

Grube, J., & Piliavin, J.A. (2000). Role identity, organizational experiences, and volunteer experiences. *Personality and Social Psychology Bulletin, 26*(9), 1108-1120.

Havighurst, R. J. (1961). Successful aging. *The Gerontologist, 1*(1), 8-13.

Havighurst, R. J., & Albrecht, R. (1953). *Older people.* New York: Longmans Green.

McAdams, D. P. (1985). *Power, intimacy, and the life story: Personological inquires into identity.* New York: Guilford Press.

McAdams, D. P., & de St. Aubin, E. (1992). A theory of generativity and its assessment through self-report, behavioral acts, and narrative themes in autobiography. *Journal of Personality and Social Psychology, 62,* 1003-1015.

Myerhoff, B. (1978). *Number our days.* New York: Simon and Schuster.

Parker, R. G. (1995). Reminiscence: A continuity theory framework. *Gerontologist, 35*(4), 515-525.

Retirement [def. 1b]. (n.d.). In *Merriam-Webster's dictionary online.* Retrieved January 3, 2013, from http://www.merriam-webster.com/dictionary/retirement?show=0&t=1392835045.

Rowe, J. W., & Kahn, R. L. (1997). Successful aging. *The Gerontologist, 37*(4), 433-440.

Shultz, K. S. (2003). Bridge employment: Work after retirement. In G. A. Adams & T.A. Beehr (Eds.), *Retirement: Reasons, processes and results* (pp. 214-241). New York: Springer Publishing Company.

Siebert, D. C., Mutran, E. J., & Reitzes, D. C. (1999). Friendship and social support: The importance of role identity to aging adults. *Social Work, 44*(6), 522-533.

Stewart, A. J., Franz, C., & Layton, L. (1988). The changing self: Using personal documents to study lives. *Journal of Personality, 56*(1), 41-74.

Stower, J., Pervewe, P. L., & Munyon, T. P. (2011). The role of identity in extra-role behaviors: Development of a conceptual model. *Journal of Managerial Psychology, 26*(2), 94-107.

Stryker, S., & Burke, P. J. (2000). The past, present, and future of an identity theory. *Social Psychology Quarterly, 63*(4), 284-97.

Stryker, S., & Statham, A. (1985). Symbolic interaction and role theory. In G. Lindzey & E. Aronson (Eds.), *The hand-book of social psychology* (pp. 311-378). New York: Random House.

Tajfel, H. (1978). Social categorization, social identity, and social comparison. In H. Tajfel (Ed.), *Differentiation between social groups: Studies in social psychology of intergroup relations* (pp. 61-76). London: Academic Press.

Trafford, A. (2004). *My time: Making the most of the rest of your life.* New York: Basic Books.

von Bonsdorff, M. E., Shultz, K. S., & Leskinen, E. (2009). The choice between retirement and bridge employment: A continuity theory and life course perspective. *International Journal of Aging and Human Development, 69*(2), 79-100.

Webster, J. D., Bohlmeijer, E. T., & Westerhof, G. J. (2010). Mapping the future of reminiscence: A conceptual guide for research and practice. *Research on Aging, 32*(4), 527-564.

4

Social Justice and the Older Worker

Susan Magasi, PhD; Denise M. Nepveux, PhD, OTR/L;
and Aimée Thompson, BSc (Hons)

Everyone has the right to work, to free choice of employment, to just and favorable conditions of work and to protection against unemployment.—United Nations, Universal Declaration of Human Rights (1948)

It has been suggested that a socially just society is one where all individuals have the right and the opportunity to participate freely in the workforce in jobs that preserve human dignity and provide economic stability (Koller, 2009; Tremblay & Genin, 2010). Economic structures and working environments have historically disadvantaged certain groups of workers based on age, gender, race/ethnicity, and disability status; often on the grounds that these groups are less fit to participate in the labor market. Advocates for social justice have fought against biological determinism, and sought to create greater equality of opportunity. In the United States, as in many other developed countries, laws such as the Equal Pay Act of 1963, the Age Discrimination in Employment Act of 1967, and the Americans with Disabilities Act of 1991 have been enacted to protect workers from discrimination. Yet, the systematic exclusion of older workers remains pervasive because attitudes and practices about work and retirement are deeply embedded in the social fabric of society.

The Madrid International Plan of Action on Ageing (MIPAA) emerged from the United Nations Second World Assembly on Ageing, and represents the commitment of over 160 governments and organizations worldwide to integrate the rights of older people into economic and social development policies within their own countries and internationally. MIPAA seeks to support and promote workforce participation by older people and ensure that they share in the benefits of economic participation and development. Despite broad-based international support for the inclusion of older people in the workforce, they face tremendous pressure, both subtle and overt, to exit the workforce.

Hunt LA, Wolverson C.
Work and the Older Person: Increasing Longevity and Well-Being (pp 37-48).
© 2015 SLACK Incorporated.

In this chapter, we will examine the social justice issues that surround older workers, including the following:

- Demographic trends in the society and in the workforce
- Policies and trends that influence older workers
- Understanding older people's motivations for work and retirement, including a discussion of differences by subgroups based on gender, race, ethnicity, and socioeconomic status
- Ageism and discrimination in the workplace

Woven throughout the chapter are considerations of political and economic factors that influence older people's workforce participation. It is also important to recognize that older workers are not a homogenous population. There are significant differences, both across subgroups based on demographic characteristics such as socioeconomic status, gender, race, ethnicity, and health status, and within groups based on personal preferences, attitudes and beliefs, and family support.

DEMOGRAPHIC TRENDS IN SOCIETY AND IN THE WORKFORCE

Since 2005, there has been an average annual population increase of 81 million people, and world populations are projected to continue to grow rapidly. People aged 60 or above are the fastest-growing segment of the population, and their numbers are expected to more than triple by 2100 (United Nations, 2013). In the United States alone, older people will account for roughly 20% of the population by 2030 (Centers for Disease Control and Prevention, 2013). Not only are more people living to old age, older people are also living longer, and life expectancies are projected to continue to increase (United Nations, 2013).

Along with the aging of the population, there has been an increase in workforce participation by older people (Heidkamp, Corre, & Van Horn, 2010). According to the Bureau of Labor Statistics, the portion of the labor force (including those who were employed or looking for employment) aged 65 and older increased by 7.1% between 1985 and 2011 (U.S. Bureau of Labor, 2013). In 2012, the number of American workers 65 and over reached 7.7 million (Rix, 2012). Demographics of the aging population alone do not account for the significant rise in employment of older workers. The graying of the Baby Boomer generation (people born between 1946 and 1964) along with economic and social trends are driving the employment rates for older workers. Throughout their lives, Baby Boomers have pushed social boundaries and transformed social structures. As they reach retirement age, this generation will have a radical impact on both work and retirement. As a group, they are healthier and better educated and have a greater sense of entitlement than previous generations. These factors influence both their expectations about work-life balance, and the economic and social resources they have as they confront the state-defined normal retirement age.

POLICIES AND TRENDS THAT INFLUENCE OLDER WORKERS

The U.S. Social Security Act of 1935 set the normal retirement age—the minimum age for receiving full retirement benefits—at 65. As life expectancies grew, the length of time between retirement and death has been extended, thereby increasing the length of time that older people have to rely on fixed incomes from Social Security and retirement savings. This shift has placed increased demands on personal retirement savings and public pension programs (Munnell, Meme, Jivan, & Cahill, 2004). To offset the economic pressures on state-sponsored pensions, and to a lesser degree, to allow older workers more time to accrue benefits, the U.S. Congress sought a gradual increase in the age for collecting full Social Security retirement benefits to 67 (Svahn & Ross, 1983). Many other industrialized countries have similarly increased their retirement age. Legislators have also sought to increase the financial security of older workers by enacting tax reform aimed at keeping more money in the hands of older workers and retirees (Friedberg, 2000). Despite efforts to delay retirement and promote workforce participation by older people, evidence suggests that age discrimination in the workforce negatively impacts older people's full and equal participation.

In 1967, the U.S. Federal Government passed the Age Discrimination in Employment Act (ADEA) to limit the deleterious impact of age discrimination in the workplace. Many individual states have supplemented the ADEA with additional state age discrimination laws. These laws have been particularly successful in reducing incidents of age discrimination in terminations, but comparative studies have shown that age discrimination, particularly related to hiring processes, remains pervasive (Adams, 2002, 2004; Johnson & Neumark, 1996; Lahey, 2008). Indeed, it has been suggested that because ADEA makes it difficult to terminate the employment of older workers, some hiring directors may be loath to hire them in the first place, thereby effectively shifting age discrimination from the firing to the hiring process (Lahey, 2008; Neumark & Song, 2011). Although scholars and economists debate the mechanism by which age discrimination in the workplace occurs, they are unanimous in their agreement that age discrimination is a reality for older workers in hiring, promotion, and retirement processes. Job loss and forced retirement are major concerns for older workers (AARP Public Policy Institute, 2012). Unemployed Boomers cited job loss as the main reason for not working (47%), followed by an "inability to find work" (19%). The "bad economy" emerged as the most difficult barrier job-seeking Boomers faced in their search for work; still, nearly 1 in 3 felt that age discrimination was the greatest barrier.

Skills obsolescence caused by rapid technological advances in the increasingly knowledge-based economy, and the failure of both older people and employers to invest in ongoing training and continuing education adversely affect older workers. Government initiatives are increasingly focusing on the development of (re)training programs that target older workers. Evidence suggests that these initiatives are underutilized, with relatively few older people taking advantage of these programs (Heidkamp et al., 2010). For example, as part of the 2009 American Recovery and Reinvestment Act (ARRA), the federal government directed $120 million to the Senior Community Service Employment Program (SCSEP), and an additional $225 million in the 2010 appropriation (U.S. Bureau of Labor, 2013). However, the SCSEP program serves less than 1% of potentially eligible clients, and outcomes data are not yet available (Heidkamp et al., 2010). Bridge and retraining programs remain attractive options in light of the continued impact of the recession of 2008 on unemployment among older workers.

According to the National Bureau of Economic Research (2010), the recession that began in December 2007 officially ended in June 2009, leaving remnants of prolonged joblessness, financial insecurity, stress, and dissatisfaction with employment in its wake. As of June 2013, there were still 11.8 million individuals in search of work. While workers of all ages were left jobless during the recession, older job seekers appear to be facing more complications finding a job than their younger counterparts (Heidkamp et al., 2010). The current rate of unemployment for older workers is low in comparison to younger workers; however, the number of workers age 55 and over experiencing unemployment has grown substantially since the recession began in 2007 (up from 3.1% at the start of the recession) (Rix, 2012). The low employment rate among seniors is indicative of slowing labor force growth relative to population, and a rising dependency ratio (Neumark & Song, 2011). Unemployment statistics may obscure the impact that the economic downturn and financial crisis has had on older people. For example, unemployed older workers were less likely to find new employment and were out of work longer than younger workers, and 84% of those older workers who were unemployed in August 2009 remained unemployed in March 2010. Older people have the highest rates of long-term unemployment; the estimated average period of unemployment for job seekers aged 55 and over is 60 weeks, compared to 38.5 weeks for younger job seekers (Rix, 2012). Many older workers were involuntarily working part-time because they could not find full-time employment, while others were becoming discouraged and leaving the labor force with the assumption that they would not find new jobs (Rix, 2012).

In addition to the rising numbers of unemployed and underemployed people and increasing duration of unemployment, the recession had a significant negative impact on the financial security of older individuals. The financial crisis led to a precipitous drop in the stock market, which effectively decimated the retirement savings of many older people. Both personal savings and public pensions were affected, causing many older people to feel that the economic safety net and carefully accrued nest eggs were snatched from them. At the same time, housing prices plummeted, limiting the value of many older people's homes, which are their most significant financial assets. A 2012 study by the AARP Public Policy Institute revealed that job loss, compensation reductions, declining home values, investment losses, and high debt have undermined retirement plans and expectations of many older workers. The shifting economic environment coupled with the graying of the Baby Boomer generation are changing the way many older people weigh decisions about retirement and work, and are leading to increasing numbers of older adults in the workforce. These numbers are shaped by personal preferences and economic necessity. To understand the social justice issues that confront older workers, it is important to recognize the personal and social factors that drive employment in later life.

UNDERSTANDING OLDER PEOPLE'S MOTIVATIONS FOR WORK AND RETIREMENT

It is not possible to talk about work and social justice without considering the material and economic reality of older workers. Ultimately, older workers must conduct a cost-benefit analysis to weigh the relative advantages of working and retirement. Interactions between the macro (state of the economy), meso (corporate and work climate), and micro (personal preferences and abilities) environments must be taken into consideration (Szinovacz, Martin, & Davey, 2013). In the next section, we will examine some of the social and environmental factors that influence older workers.

The Baby Boomer generation is redefining aging. They are healthier and better educated and have a greater sense of entitlement than previous generations, including expectations about work-life balance and active retirement. An AARP study (2004) found that 80% of Baby Boomers plan to keep working, in some capacity, until at least 65 (AARP, 2004). A growing number of older people, both by choice and by necessity, plan to continue to work at least part-time after the traditional retirement age. In fact, many older people find the prospect of retirement unattractive, and forced retirement policies are widely unpopular. At the same time, policies that seek to raise the age of eligibility for retirement benefits and essentially force older workers to remain in the workforce are also viewed with resentment (Tremblay & Genin, 2010).

Inherent in the discussion about working late is the presumption of choice. As we consider the choices that individuals make, we must also consider the market and economic realities in which people live. Arguably, the opportunities available to older workers are shaped by market forces, as well as decisions and opportunities available to them across the life span (Laws, 1995; McMullin & Marshall, 2001). Let us consider a few examples about how subgroup differences may influence the choices and opportunities of older workers.

Low-wage workers who have worked two jobs just to make a living may face different social justice issues than older executives fighting to retain seats on the board of directors. A secure retirement may be beyond the reach of some older workers who continue to toil in low-wage and often physically demanding jobs. Similarly, older women may be a particularly vulnerable subgroup of older workers. Many older women have intermittent work histories because of caregiving responsibilities or adherence to traditional gender roles (i.e., full-time homemaker). As a result, they may have accrued fewer retirement benefits, placing them at risk for poverty later in life, especially those living alone due to widowhood or divorce. The combination of the need to work to supplement fixed incomes with limited work histories may restrict their employment and retirement choices. Finally, older workers' expectations and sense of entitlement may factor into their choices for second and bridge-to-retirement careers. Considerations may include the type of work and the salary range deemed acceptable. For example, autoworkers who took early retirement may have expectations based on their history of strong union representation, long-term employment, and specialized skills that enabled them to earn a high salary in the manufacturing industry. These skills and corresponding salary and status expectations may not translate to the new economy, with its emphasis on service and information technologies (D. McKay, personal communication, July 18, 2013).

In order to understand the social justice issues that influence older workers, it is important to recognize that different groups of workers may experience different motivations and different social pressures when it comes to work and retirement. Through better understanding of the needs of diverse groups of workers, organizations (both business and government) can better support older people who want to continue to work, those who want to scale back, and those who want to permanently exit the workforce.

The most obvious reason that people work is to make money, either for economic survival or to maintain a certain quality of life and standard of living (Evans et al., 2008). Increasingly, older workers rely on their income to support not only themselves, but also adult children and grandchildren (Pienta & Hayward, 2002). The desire to pass wealth along to future generations has been identified as a primary retirement planning and investment goal, especially among people of racial minority communities (ING Retirement Research Institute, 2012; Prudential Research Institute, 2013). Maintenance of health insurance and the continued accrual of work-related benefits were also cited as important reasons to continue working. Older workers also value the independence that working affords them.

Rapid and unexpected losses of personal wealth in the recession of 2008 imposed new pressures on workers facing retirement (Szinovacz, Martin, & Davey, 2013). The economic pressure simultaneously forced some older workers to postpone retirement, while presenting unemployed or underemployed older workers with very limited opportunities to find new employment. It may also have forced some workers out of the labor market against their will (Coile & Levine, 2007, 2011). Research has shown that the terms of a person's retirement have significant impact on long-term outcomes, with older workers who perceive that their retirement was forced having much poorer health and quality of life (Bender, 2012; Hershey & Henkens, 2013). Szinovacz and Davey (2004) found that nearly one-third of older workers perceived that their retirement was forced by poor health, job displacement, and care obligations. Older workers with higher socioeconomic status have significantly greater choice about work and retirement. Paradoxically, despite fewer retirement resources and accumulated benefits, women, people with less education, and workers from racial and ethnic minority groups are more likely to retire early (Aaron & Callan, 2011; McGarry, 2004). For example, Blacks are more likely to exit the workforce earlier (possibly because of limited opportunities and tendency to occupy low-wage, physically demanding jobs), but have less retirement savings than their White counterparts. In fact, although Blacks contribute a larger percentage of their paychecks to retirement plans, the actual dollar amount contributed is significantly lower ($157 vs. $220 overall; ING Retirement Research Institute, 2012). Both Blacks and Hispanics are more likely to have caregiving responsibilities and to be supporting other people financially than the general population. High debt is cited as the biggest barrier to saving for retirement, especially among Black women. Similarly, Latino/Hispanic workers tend to have lower retirement savings (both in employer-sponsored and personal retirement plans) than either non-Hispanic Whites or Blacks. Reasons for not investing in retirement saving plans include inadequate income to meet day-to-day expenses, high debt, and lack of knowledge about investment opportunities. According to economists, racial, ethnic, and gender differences in retirement plan participation are related to life course differences in work histories, social and economic (dis)advantages, health, and human capital, rather than inherent to the retirement planning process itself (Flippen & Tienda, 2000;

Szinovacz & Davey, 2004). While perhaps not causally related to retirement decisions, those concerned with social justice and work must pay closer attention to the long-term impact that working conditions now will have on the older workers of tomorrow.

In addition to the economic benefits of work, research has shown that older people value participation in the workforce because it contributes to their self-concept and thus allows them to maintain a sense of meaning in their lives (Atchley, 1989). For many adults, lifelong engagement in a particular career or profession is a defining part of who they are, and the ability to maintain that identity is highly valued (see Chapter 3 for a detailed discussion of the Purposeful Aging Theory). Indeed, passion for the work itself reinforces older peoples' commitments to employment (Fraser, McKenna, Turpin, Allen, & Liddle, 2009). Work has also been identified as a means of giving back to the community. Giving back may be accomplished in a variety of ways, including mentoring younger workers and providing important links to the company's history. There is an increasing trend among older workers to transition from full-time employment to bridge careers with a public service orientation. Bridge careers, once seen as a privilege of the upper classes, are now identified with people at both the higher and lower ends of the wage distribution (Cahill, Giandrea, & Quinn, 2006). Erikson's construct of generativity, once thought to be a pursuit of people 40 to 65, clearly persists well beyond the traditional age of retirement. Indeed, many older people, both workers and retirees, seek opportunities for civic engagement in and outside of the labor market as a way to give back to others (Kaskie, Imhof, Cavanaugh, & Culp, 2008). From social justice and economic opportunity perspectives, it is important not to relegate older workers to the roles of free laborers and volunteers, or to neglect their material needs (Martinson & Minkler, 2006). Finally, for many older people, the workplace represents an important space for socialization and social engagement (Bambrick & Bonder, 2005).

In the discussion of social justice and older workers, it is important to recognize that retirement remains an attractive and desired option for many people. Retirement is seen by many as both a right and a reward that one earns at the end of a long work life (Tremblay & Genin, 2010). In fact, early retirement is frequently touted as a sign of personal prosperity and financial success. For example, Tremblay et al. found that 40% of people surveyed plan to retire before the age of 55. Another third of workers plan to retire between 65 and 69. The reality is that work and retirement are not dichotomous variables in the lives of older people. Older workers express a preference for flexibility in scheduling, work hours, and retirement strategies (Tremblay & Genin, 2010).

AGEISM AND DISCRIMINATION IN THE WORKPLACE

Ageism is a form of discrimination based on stereotypic attitudes and the social devaluation of older people (Butler, 1969). Although ageism is prevalent in today's society, it may be more difficult to detect than other forms of discrimination (Rupp, Vodanovich, & Credé, 2005). Ageism in the workforce can lead to overt discrimination, social exclusion, and mistreatment of older workers (Brownell & Kelly, 2013). Some consequences of ageism in the workforce are harassment of older workers, exclusionary policies, and denial of opportunities in hiring, training and retention. Ageism and age discrimination are pervasive in the workplace. Over 81% of older workers in the United States had experienced workplace discrimination within the past year (Chou & Choi, 2011).

The International Longevity Center (2008) has identified four overlapping types of ageism that may affect older workers (International Longevity Center, 2008). *Personal ageism* refers to negative attitudes and practices that individuals have towards older people, as a group and as individuals. Examples may include avoiding the grocery store checkout line with the 60-year-old cashier because of assumptions that she will be slower than her younger colleagues, or excluding an older colleague from a brainstorming session on a new marketing campaign because of the belief that older workers are less creative and less able to cope with the demands of a tight deadline. Older people are not immune to ageism and may internalize these negative attitudes about their own worth and productivity in the workforce (Levy, 2003; Maurer, 2001; McMullin & Marshall, 2001).

The past two decades have seen a proliferation of media and public service campaigns emphasizing healthy and active aging. The healthy aging paradigm sought to counteract ageist stereotypes against older people. AARP has been at the forefront of these campaigns, which highlight attractive, smiling older people engaged in a wide range of active pursuits, such as biking, golfing, and dancing. The underlying message of such campaigns is that if you work hard, invest well, and take control of your health, the fruits of active aging can be yours. Healthy aging has become a moral imperative and a personal responsibility; consequently, it may have a perverse effect on people who—because of lack of opportunity, social and environmental inequities, or medical "bad luck"—experience age-related functional loss, social isolation, and economic deprivation. People may internalize these beliefs and devalue older people who fall short of the healthy aging ideal—a devaluation that may play out in the workforce.

Institutional ageism is the systematic exclusion of individuals or groups based on age. This exclusion is embedded in the programs, policies, and practices of the workplace. Institutional ageism may occur at the work site, (e.g., when companies systematically fail to retrain older workers as new technologies are adopted) or when older workers are scheduled for all the weekend or evening shifts because of the belief that, as empty nesters, they lack childcare responsibilities. Not only do such beliefs relegate older people to less desirable shifts, they also ignore the important roles that many older people play as unpaid caregivers to spouses, grandchildren, and, in some instances, to their own elder parents. Institutional ageism is also embedded in social and governmental structures and policies. For example, age-based pension and benefit programs pressure older workers to exit the workforce to make room for younger workers by accepting severance packages and early retirement during corporate downsizing. Union policies have been shown to be biased in favor of younger workers (Burnay, 2010; MacGregor, 2006).

Ageism may be intentional or inadvertent. *Intentional ageism* occurs when biases against older people are knowingly translated into practice (e.g., when hiring managers refuse to interview or hire older workers). Although it is illegal in the United States and Canada to ask job seekers questions about their age, there are many clues in the application and hiring process that can tip potential employers off to an applicant's age. High school and college graduation dates and employment histories that include dates and years of experience provide potential employers with information that can bias hiring decisions. In fact, job counselors now encourage all workers, and older ones in particular, to remove dates and lengthy employment histories from their resumés and applications, lest potential employers be biased by preconceptions about salary demands, declining productivity, rising health insurance costs, or other ageist beliefs (D. McKay, personal communication, July 18, 2013).

Extensive research has documented how the media exploits ageist stereotypes. Images of the crone, the curmudgeon, and the out-of-date fuddy-duddy unable to program the latest technological gadgets are pervasive in advertising, movies, and television. The impact of these images spills over to the work world and leads to inadvertent perpetuation of ageism and age discrimination (Adams, 2002; Roscigno, 2007). *Inadvertent ageism* occurs when people and policies unwittingly disadvantage individuals or groups based on their age. Examples include situations in which employers fail to implement universal design features or reasonable accommodations for older workers into the work environment, such as larger print fonts for reports or operating manuals. Professional meetings are often held in convention centers with morning until evening schedules, typically requiring a lot of walking and extended periods sitting in uncomfortable chairs with poor ergonomic designs. Such programming can discourage participation among older people, especially those with age-related mobility and physical impairments. Inadvertent ageist practices are not implemented to harm older adults, but rather without considering the needs of a diverse workforce.

As with other racial, ethnic, and disability minority groups, language matters greatly, both as a shaper and a reflector of attitudes. Derogatory terms and jokes about older people can foster an ageist work environment and lead to devaluation, discrimination, and mistreatment of older workers. Even seemingly innocuous comments such as, "My generation is really great with technology" create intergenerational tension and subtle discrimination.

Ageism in the workplace has been shown to have a negative impact on both individuals and organizations. Ageism translates into age discriminatory practices in the hiring, training, promotion, and retention process. At the individual level, age discriminatory practices can lead to decreased self-efficacy, decreased performance, and even cardiovascular stress (Levy, Ashman, & Dror, 2000; Levy, Hausdorff, Hencke, & Wei, 2000).

Age discrimination does not only affect workers. With a median award of $268,926 and recent multimillion dollar settlements, discrimination law suits based on ageism can also be costly for employers (Rupp et al., 2005).

CASE STUDY

The following case study illustrates how life course experiences and limited investment in older workers can negatively impact older workers' job satisfaction, health, and prospects for continued involvement in the workforce.

Lautaro, a 63-year-old man of South American origin, was in his first year of university when his country's government fell to a right-wing coup in the mid-1970s. As a union representative who was active in the political left, he fled the country and emigrated to Canada as a political refugee.

Early Work Life
In his youth, Lautaro worked low-wage jobs in a variety of industries, including the garment industry, auto plants, and nickel mines and refineries. These jobs were characterized by inhospitable work environments, including high stress, poor health and safety standards, and a sense of alienation from his coworkers based on linguistic and cultural differences. He had little job security and was laid off several times. The combination of poor working conditions and job stress caused him to become physically ill and his health remains fragile as a result. Despite job dissatisfaction, he found fulfillment in civic engagement and political activism. He began pursuing a path out of factory work by doing janitorial work at night and taking courses during the day. He earned a diploma in television broadcasting. He had to take temporary low-skilled jobs, such as duplicating videotapes, but his dream was to write, produce, and direct meaningful television programs.

Finally, in his early 40s, Lautaro landed a permanent job at a local TV station. The company's director was a visionary who drove broadcast innovations and emphasized that TV broadcasting should reflect the diversity of Canada. Lautaro was pleased to be working in such a company and was promoted to Master Control Operator.

Lautaro made responsible decisions to ensure his financial security, including avoiding debt and purchasing a small condo near to his workplace. He did not marry, have children, or own a car. Although Lautaro's job title has remained the same for the past 20 years, many aspects of the job have changed around him and have affected his career, lifestyle, and well-being.

Corporatization and Technological Change
When Lautaro started, he was working with analog technology (videotapes) and little was automated. He worked with other operators to ensure that the channel's content flowed

smoothly and continuously. Gradually, the network expanded to include more channels. The pace and mental demands of the work escalated as more of the technology became digitized and automated, and operators were asked to monitor multiple channels simultaneously.

Expertise that was previously valued was rendered obsolete. Although the pace of technological and software upgrades accelerated, the company's investment in training plummeted. Lautaro is expected to self-train via tutorials and manuals. Operators are blamed for problems that they have received little training to rectify. Lautaro sees the company's rapid adoption of technology as an effort to eliminate his position altogether. His employers have not invested in his education. His knowledge of computers is limited, and his ambition to pursue further education has been limited by shift work. His college training has become outmoded. He sees no option other than to remain in his position until retirement, and then perhaps to pursue a part-time job as a laborer or building security guard.

Long-Term Impact of Shift Work

Twenty years of shift work have taken a toll on Lautaro's physical and social well-being. He is keenly aware that a rotating schedule, isolation on the job, 12-hour shifts, and poor sleep affect long-term health. Shift work has diminished Lautaro's opportunities to engage socially and build social networks. He has a small circle of loyal friends, but feels somewhat lonely and isolated, often missing holidays and social occasions because of his work schedule. His unpredictable schedule also makes it hard for him to pursue opportunities for civic engagement or personal development.

Barriers to Mobility and Promotion

Lautaro has retained the Master Control Operator position through several mergers, buyouts, and mass layoffs. He has applied for other positions within the company, and believes that his skills and seniority merit consideration, but he has never received serious consideration. He feels trapped in the literal and figurative "basement" of the company— a permanent entry level to which colleagues may descend when layoffs occur, but from which no one is allowed to advance. He advises younger colleagues to find other jobs as soon as possible, and not get "stuck in the basement."

Through mergers and buyouts, the positive and egalitarian work culture that Lautaro valued has been lost. The employment context has also changed. Provincial antidiscrimination protections—important to Lautaro as an immigrant and a person of color—were dismantled in 1995 under the Harris government, in favor of looser "diversity" policies (Bakan & Kobayashi, 2007).

Retirement Prospects

At 63, Lautaro is in fairly good health, notwithstanding back pain and other chronic issues that he is actively managing. He owns his home outright, is debt free, and has retirement savings. He hopes to retire, or at least reduce his employment and cease shift work, at 65. He hopes to pursue education and travel, perhaps taking a voluntary service position abroad. He has never received financial counseling and is unsure how realistic his hopes may be.

Summary

Lautaro's story is emblematic of the plight of many low-skilled and low-wage older workers and immigrants. Early work experiences, including limited social support, unstable work history, and job transience forced him into a job with limited opportunities for professional advancement or personal fulfillment. The work world has changed around him, including the corporatization of his workplace. Rapidly changing technologies have hindered job satisfaction and limited his job market prospects. As a result of an unfulfilling work life, Lautaro is eager to leave his company, but worries that skills obsolescence will limit his alternatives for part-time work. Lautaro has the advantage that due to lifelong financial prudence, he has the resources to support his retirement. However, due to a lack of active retirement planning, he is uncertain as to whether his means are sufficient to allow him to achieve his retirement dreams.

CONCLUSION

Keeping older workers employed longer is an important issue, especially from a social justice perspective. Social justice principles can increase both efficiency and productivity in the workplace (Koller, 2009; Tremblay, 2010). It is recommended that employers adopt practices to encourage older workers to remain in the workforce. Employers should identify and reduce ageist practices, both inadvertent and intentional, to create an environment in which older workers are supported and valued. This can include the purposeful inclusion of age-related issues into corporate diversity initiatives and cultural competency trainings. Employers should integrate universal design principles into the physical and built environment and into information and communication technologies to mitigate the impact that age-related functional decline has on job-related tasks. Employers should invest equally in older workers, especially in the areas of retraining and continuing education, to ensure that older workers' skills continue to evolve and keep pace with technological advances and job demands. To help better prepare older workers for their eventual exit from the workforce, improved financial education and retirement planning opportunities should be made available to all workers regardless of age. These efforts should be tailored to the needs and priorities of different subgroups of workers (e.g., women, minority group members). Finally, workers at different life stages may have different priorities and needs when trying to balance their work and personal lives. The implementation of flexibility and customizability into scheduling and planning of work hours, job tasks, and exit strategies can help accommodate the diverse needs and priorities of older workers.

Ageism and age discrimination in the workforce are social justice issues because they unfairly limit older people's employment opportunities. These include not only opportunities to find and maintain work, but also opportunities for advancement, training, and promotion. Restricted opportunities may force many older people into retirement, which can negatively impact their financial security, health, and quality of life. Equal opportunities for employment should be made available to all older people—both those who want to work and those who need to work.

REFERENCES

Aaron, H. J., & Callan, J. M. (2011). *Who retires early?* Boston College Center for Retirement Research Working Paper.

AARP. (2004). *Baby Boomers envision retirement II.* Washington, DC: American Association of Retired Persons.

AARP Public Policy Institute. (2012). *Boomers and the great recession: Struggling to recover.* Washington, DC: American Association of Retired Persons.

Adams, S. J. (2002). Passed over for promotion because of age: An empirical analysis of the consequences. *Journal of Labor Research, 23*(3), 447-461.

Adams, S. J. (2004). Age discrimination legislation and the employment of older workers. *Labour Economics, 11*(2), 219-241.

Atchley, R. C. (1989). A continuity theory of normal aging. *The Gerontologist, 29*(2), 183-190.

Bakan, A. B., & Kobayashi, A. (2007). 'The sky didn't fall': Organizing to combat racism in the workplace—The case of the Alliance for Employment Equity. In G. F. Johnson & R. Enomoto (Eds.), *Race, Racialization and Antiracism in Canada and Beyond.* Toronto: University of Toronto Press.

Bambrick, P., & Bonder, B. (2005). Older adults' perceptions of work. *Work: A Journal of Prevention, Assessment and Rehabilitation, 24*(1), 77-84.

Bender, K. A. (2012). An analysis of well-being in retirement: The role of pensions, health, and 'voluntariness' of retirement. *The Journal of Socio-Economics, 41*(4), 424-433.

Brownell, P., & Kelly, J. J. (Eds.). (2013). *Ageism and Mistreatment of Older Workers: Current Reality, Future Solutions.* New York: Springer.

Burnay, N. (2010). Older workers in changing social policy patterns. *Studies in Social Justice, 3*(2), 155-171.

Business Cycle Dating Committee, National Bureau of Economic Research. (2010). Retrieved July 5 2010, from http://www.nber.org/cycles/sept2010.html.

Butler, R. N. (1969). Age-ism: Another form of bigotry. *The Gerontologist, 9*(4 Part 1), 243-246.

Cahill, K. E., Giandrea, M. D., & Quinn, J. F. (2006). Retirement patterns from career employment. *The Gerontologist, 46*(4), 514-523.

Centers for Disease Control and Prevention. (2013). *The state of aging and health in America 2013.* Atlanta, GA: CDC.

Chou, R. J.-A., & Choi, N. G. (2011). Prevalence and correlates of perceived workplace discrimination among older workers in the United States of America. *Ageing and Society, 31*(6), 1051.

Coile, C. C., & Levine, P. B. (2007). Labor market shocks and retirement: Do government programs matter? *Journal of Public Economics, 91*(10), 1902-1919.

Coile, C. C., & Levine, P. B. (2011). The market crash and mass layoffs: How the current economic crisis may affect retirement. *The BE Journal of Economic Analysis & Policy, 11*(1), 22.

Evans, D. M., Conte, K., Gilroy, M., Marvin, T., Theysohn, H., & Fisher, G. (2008). Occupational therapy–Meeting the needs of older adult workers? *Work: A Journal of Prevention, Assessment and Rehabilitation, 31*(1), 73-82.

Flippen, C., & Tienda, M. (2000). Pathways to retirement: Patterns of labor force participation and labor market exit among the pre-retirement population by race, Hispanic origin, and sex. *Journals of Gerontology Series B, 55*(1), S14-S27.

Fraser, L., McKenna, K., Turpin, M., Allen, S., & Liddle, J. (2009). Older workers: An exploration of the benefits, barriers and adaptations for older people in the workforce. *Work: A Journal of Prevention, Assessment and Rehabilitation, 33*(3), 261-272.

Friedberg, L. (2000). The labor supply effects of the social security earnings test. *Review of Economics and Statistics, 82*(1), 48-63.

Heidkamp, M., Corre, N., & Van Horn, C. E. (2010). The 'new unemployables': Older job seekers struggle to find work during the great recession. *The Sloan Center on Aging Work at Boston College.* Available at: https://www.bc.edu/content/dam/files/research_sites/agingandwork/pdf/publications/IB25_NewUnemployed.pdf.

Hershey, D. A., & Henkens, K. (2014). Impact of different types of retirement transitions on perceived satisfaction with life. *The Gerontologist, 54*(2), 232-244.

ING Retirement Research Institute. (2012). Culture complex: Examining the retirement and financial habits, attitudes and preparedness of America's diverse workforce. New York, NY.

International Longevity Center. (2008). *Ageism in America.* New York: Open Society Institute.

Johnson, R. W., & Neumark, D. (1996). Age discrimination, job separation, and employment status of older workers: Evidence from self-reports. *Journal of Human Resources, 32*(4), 779-811.

Kaskie, B., Imhof, S., Cavanaugh, J., & Culp, K. (2008). Civic engagement as a retirement role for aging Americans. *The Gerontologist, 48*(3), 368-377.

Koller, P. (2009). Work and social justice. *Analyse & Kritik, 31*(1), 5-24.

Lahey, J. (2008). State age protection laws and the age discrimination in employment act. *Journal of Law and Economics, 51*(3), 433-460.

Laws, G. (1995). Understanding ageism: Lessons from feminism and postmodernism. *The Gerontologist, 35*(1), 112-118.

Levy, B., Ashman, O., & Dror, I. (2000). To be or not to be: The effects of aging stereotypes on the will to live. *Omega (Westport), 40*(3), 409-420.

Levy, B., Hausdorff, J. M., Hencke, R., & Wei, J. Y. (2000). Reducing cardiovascular stress with positive self-stereotypes of aging. *The Journals of Gerontology Series B:Psychological Sciences and Social Sciences, 55*(4), P205-P213.

Levy, B. R. (2003). Mind matters: Cognitive and physical effects of aging self-stereotypes. *The Journals of Gerontology Series B: Psychological Sciences and Social Sciences, 58*(4), P203-P211.

MacGregor, D. (2006). Editorial: neglecting elders in the workplace: civil society organizations, ageism, and mandatory retirement. *Canadian Journal on Aging, 25*(3), 243-246.

Martinson, M., & Minkler, M. (2006). Civic engagement and older adults: A critical perspective. *The Gerontologist, 46*(3), 318-324.

Maurer, T. J. (2001). Career-relevant learning and development, worker age, and beliefs about self-efficacy for development. *Journal of Management, 27*(2), 123-140.

McGarry, K. (2004). Health and retirement: Do changes in health affect retirement expectations? *Journal of Human Resources, 39*(3), 624-648.

McMullin, J. A., & Marshall, V. W. (2001). Ageism, age relations, and garment industry work in Montreal. *The Gerontologist, 41*(1), 111-122.

Munnell, A., Meme, K., Jivan, N., & Cahill, K. (2004). Should we raise Social Security's earliest eligibility age? Center for Retirement Research at Boston College. Retrieved January 3, 2013, from http://crr.bc.edu/briefs/should-we-raise-social-securitys-earliest-eligibility-age/.

Neumark, D., & Song, J. (2011). Do stronger age discrimination laws make Social Security reforms more effective? National Bureau of Economic Research. Retrieved January 3, 2014, from http://www.nber.org/papers/w17467.

Pienta, A. M., & Hayward, M. D. (2002). Who expects to continue working after age 62? The retirement plans of couples. *The Journals of Gerontology Series B: Psychological Sciences and Social Sciences, 57*(4), S199-S208.

Prudential Research Institute. (2013). *The African American financial experience: 2013-2014.* Newark, NJ: Prudential Research.

Rix, S. (2012). The employment situation, April 2012: Little encouraging news for older adults. Washington, D.C.: AARP. Retrieved from http://www.aarp.org/content/dam/aarp/research/public_policy_institute/econ_sec/2012/The-Employment-Situation-April-2012-AARP-ppi-econ-sec.pdf.

Roscigno, V. J., Mong, S., Byron, R., & Tester, G. (2007). Age discrimination, social closure and employment. *Social Forces, 86*(1), 313-334.

Rupp, D. E., Vodanovich, S. J., & Credé, M. (2005). The multidimensional nature of ageism: Construct validity and group differences. *The Journal of Social Psychology, 145*(3), 335-362.

Svahn, J. A., & Ross, M. (1983). Social Security Amendments of 1983: Legislative history and summary of provisions. *Soc. Sec. Bull., 46*, 3.

Szinovacz, M., Martin, L., & Davey, A. (2013). Recession and expected retirement age: Another look at the evidence. *The Gerontologist, 54*(2), 245-257

Szinovacz, M. E., & Davey, A. (2004). Retirement transitions and spouse disability: Effects on depressive symptoms. *The Journals of Gerontology: Series B: Psychological Sciences and Social Sciences, 59*(6), S333-S342.

Tremblay, D.-G. (2010). Work, insecurity, and social justice. *Studies in Social Justice, 3*(2), 145-154.

Tremblay, D.-G., & Genin, É. (2010). Aging, economic insecurity, and employment: Which measures would encourage older workers to stay longer in the labor market? *Studies in Social Justice, 3*(2), 173-190.

U.S. Bureau of Labor. (2013). Employment Situation Summary-June 2013.

United Nations. (1948). The Universal Declaration of Human Rights. *UN News Center.* Retrieved June 4, 2014, from http://www.un.org/en/documents/udhr/.

United Nations. (2013). World Population Prospects: The 2012 Revision, Key Findings and Advance Tables *Working Paper No. ESA/P/WP.227.* New York: United Nations, Department of Economic and Social Affairs-Population Division.

5

Aging, Disability, and Work

Nancy E. Krusen, PhD, OTR/L; Linda A. Hunt, PhD, OTR/L, FAOTA; and Caroline Wolverson, DipCOT, DipHT, MSc

Work is healthy, you can hardly put more upon a man than he can bear. It is not work that kills men; it is worry. Worry is rust upon the blade.—Henry Ward Beecher (1895)

The intersection of aging, disability, and work raises a complex set of issues for which there is no single applicable paradigm. At least three distinct groups of people face direct challenges described by this chapter (Heidkamp, Mabe, & DeGraaf, 2012). The first group consists of those who have lived with a disability since early in life. They may be familiar with available resources, including technology, modifications, benefits, and accommodations. As they grow older, they may deal with the development of secondary conditions or the effects of natural aging that alter their functional abilities. The second group of people consists of individuals who acquire a physical disability as a side effect of aging. Life inevitably modifies the body, leading to physical or mechanical limitations, such as decreased mobility, hearing, or vision. Conditions such as arthritis, Parkinsonism, stroke, cancer, or heart disease often accompany the process of growing older. In addition, there are those whose disability is a result of sensory loss. The third group includes people who may have cognitive or emotional changes, such as dementia and depression. A fourth group of people who are indirectly affected by the challenges of disability and aging are family members and caregivers. Their paid work may be affected as their role changes to encompass that of caregiver. Only the first group of people may be familiar with the existing resources. Individuals who acquire a disability at a later age, have a cognitive limitation, or are affected by the disability of a family member may lack the knowledge necessary to gain or maintain safe, productive work.

Recent improvements in health care and increased life expectancy mean that many people are able to maintain both a good quality of life and a meaningful contribution to the workforce while living into old age. More workers than ever before are participating in the labor force during their later years, whether or not they age with a long-term condition. In the United States, the number of workers age 55 and older is expected to increase by 47% during the period from 2006 to 2016 (Toossi, 2007). This demographic trend is found in other Western countries. Because incidence

Hunt LA, Wolverson C.
Work and the Older Person: Increasing Longevity and Well-Being (pp 49-62).
© 2015 SLACK Incorporated.

and prevalence of disability increases with age (Stock & Beegle, 2004), it is important to examine the influence of these factors on life and work. This chapter examines both growing older with a disability acquired as a younger person, and disabilities acquired as part of the natural aging process. Through narratives, this chapter discusses the impact of aging and disability on the lives and work of people from different countries who have a lifelong disability, an acquired disability, or who are affected by the need to support someone with a disability.

DEFINITION OF AGING AND DISABILITY

There are many commonly used definitions of old age, varying with chronology, health, function, social norms, or eligibility for pension. For simplicity, this chapter uses the United Nations cutoff of 60+ years (United Nations, 2006). There is no common definition of "disability," though there are some similarities across countries. The United Nations Convention on the Rights of Persons with Disabilities specifies that disabilities arise from a combination of conditions and environmental barriers. "Persons with disabilities include those who have long-term physical, mental, intellectual or sensory impairments which in interaction with various barriers may hinder their full and effective participation in society on an equal basis with others" (United Nations, 2006). In the United States, disabilities are defined by the Americans with Disabilities Act 1990, Amended (ADA, 2009) as the following:

- A physical or mental impairment that substantially limits one or more major life activities of such individual

- A record of such an impairment

- Being regarded as having such an impairment

In the United Kingdom, the Equality Act (2010) defines disability as having a physical or mental impairment, with the impairment having a substantial and long-term adverse effect on the ability to carry out normal day-to-day activities. The Australian Government specifies disability as "one or more of 17 identified limitations, restrictions or impairments which have lasted or are likely to last, for a period of six months or more, and which restrict a person's everyday activities" (Australian Institute of Health and Welfare, 2008, para. 1).

AGING AND DISABILITY LEGISLATION

In the natural course of aging, some functional limitations will occur and may meet these definitions of disability. These limitations may decrease capacity, and potentially, decrease a worker's ability to perform specific tasks. Historically, researchers have shown that employers perceive older workers, with or without disabilities, as unable to meet high-pressure demands and long hours of work. In some instances, older workers have been bypassed for new work opportunities or were at risk of being phased out of work (Carnoy 2000; McFarlin, Song, & Sonntag, 1991). Most Western countries have enacted laws that discourage age and disability discrimination, whether based on perceived or actual performance (McMullin & Shuey 2006). The Americans with Disabilities Act (1990) is a civil rights law intended to prohibit discrimination against persons with disabilities. This law addresses employment, public transportation, public accommodations, and communication (ADA, 2009). The first Title of the Act prohibits "private employers, state and local governments, employment agencies and labor unions from discriminating against qualified individuals with disabilities." The stated prohibition pertains to job applications, hiring and firing, promotion, compensation, job training, and other terms of employment. Also in the United States, the Age Discrimination and Employment Act protects the right to work for people who are 40 years of age or older, prohibiting discrimination on the basis of age (U.S. Equal Employment Opportunity Commission, 1967).

The National Strategy for an Ageing Australia (Strategy) was implemented by the government in 2001. The Strategy is a coordinated national response to issues of population aging, outlining a framework of short-, medium-, and long-term plans for the management of challenges and opportunities presented by an older Australia. Plans include employment for older workers, deferred retirement, independence, and self-provision. The new Strategy targets flexible and broad services, and improving links between different sectors of government (National Strategy for an Ageing Australia, 2000).

In December 2012, the Australian state and territorial governments agreed on a new National Disability Insurance Scheme. The coverage will provide choice and control over care with support to families and caregivers, abolishing the current lottery system of selection (National Disability Insurance Scheme, 2012). Also in late 2012, the Australian government made several legislative changes to support workers. Changes include giving employer incentives to hire older workers, lifting limitations on worker compensation benefits, and the appointment of an Age Discrimination Commissioner for oversight of the program.

In 1995, the introduction of the Disability Discrimination Act (DDA) in Britain included requirements for employers to make "reasonable adjustments" for the removal of barriers to workers' access and participation. This included the provision of assistive devices and equipment in the workplace (where needed). The DDA was amended in 2005, and recently revised and included in the Equality Act (2010), which includes equal access to employment, regardless of both age and disability.

Absent from existing definitions of disability are functional changes resulting from the natural aging process. Whether the effects of aging ought to be addressed in disability legislation is a subject for current debate. Workers and employers may assume that a limitation is simply a result of the natural aging process. Modifications can be made to ameliorate performance deterioration in many circumstances, but if a worker does not identify or declare a disability at any age, then accommodations are not made. Both employer and worker must ascribe limitations in function to a specific, identifiable disability in order for antidiscrimination legislation to be applicable. Despite historically negative views of older workers and persons with disabilities as less capable workers, more recent literature shows that experienced workers offer task familiarity and expertise, increasing their value as employees (Haight, 2003). Employee benefit policy analysts recommend that workers in the United States should remain in the workplace longer, retiring at older ages (Turner, 2008). Jeszeck et al. (2007) describe a system of accommodation in the Netherlands, with services for older workers that parallel services for workers with disabilities.

Lifelong Disability—Australia

Jannetje is a woman in her early 60s who lives with her husband on rural farmland along the eastern coast in Australia. Jannetje had polio as a young girl. She uses a cane to walk and is developing arthritis as she ages. Jannetje has been a full-time employee throughout her adult life. Now she and her husband own their own business. Her story describes how a lifelong condition and aging affect her work and life.

A couple of years ago, my husband and I moved to the country to make a go of sustainable farming. Permaculture has been a dream of ours for a long time. My husband and I plan organic farming projects for other people and show them what to do. My husband is qualified in permaculture design. I teach life skills classes for sustainability and self-reliance. I show people how to repair things that are broken so they don't just throw them in the rubbish. I used to work at a desk. I never expected to be a farmer, but here I am. We want people to know about food and where it comes from and how to grow their own food.

I worked in an office for years but that was just my day job. It paid the bills. I am an artist and have a studio at home where I paint, mostly oils. I work in all different media. I sculpt. I still have my studio. It seems like my hands are always dirty doing something.

Jannetje describes her health care needs as having been "mostly" covered through Australia's public health care service, Medicare. Unlike the U.S. Medicare system, which is specific to elders, the Australian Medicare system funds free health care for all its citizens, including universal access to public hospital treatment. Australian Medicare is funded through a levy on taxpayers with incomes above a threshold amount. Some out-of-hospital medical treatment is subsidized and some services must be paid privately, such as dentistry, optometry, and emergency transport (Australian Government Department of Human Services, 2012). Individuals may also purchase private health insurance to cover out-of-pocket expenses or to cover faster treatment within a private facility. Jannetje and her husband have used both national and private services, depending on their health needs at the time.

I had polio when I was a little girl. It never stopped me, though. I even used to water ski. I never saw myself as "disabled." When I first met my husband, he would pick me up on his motorcycle and we would go adventuring. Since I have gotten older, there are some things I can't do. I have not had the late effects of polio you hear about but I do have arthritis. Maybe it's the same thing. I had an ankle fused and I had to have knee surgery a few years ago. Now I use a Segway for long distances instead of walking. My shoulders hurt, so I cut my hair short. I was sad but it is so much easier to take care of and I don't have to ask my husband for help. I get tired more than I used to but I can still do what I want.

In Australia, people aged 55 to 64 years with disabilities have the lowest labor market participation of all the age groups (Australian Bureau of Statistics, 2010). Jannetje does not perceive herself as disabled, despite aging with a lifelong condition that meets the definition of disability presented by the Australian Institute of Health and Welfare. She has not used income support or support services. She does say that she is fortunate that polio only affected her legs and that she has the use of her hands. She has learned efficiencies and modifications to do the things she wants to do. Jannetje is slightly older than her husband and hopes that if she needs help while aging that the changes in the new National Disability Insurance Scheme will mean that her husband will not bear the burden of caring for her. She is currently self-employed and continues to work steadily, with no plans to retire soon.

ACQUIRED PHYSICAL DISABILITY—UNITED STATES

Owen is 55 and lives in the central United States. Owen joined the military following college. After several years, he moved to a private software development company. At age 48, he was diagnosed with amyotrophic lateral sclerosis (ALS). This degenerative neuromuscular disease damages motor nerves, causing severe and progressive muscle weakness affecting the arms, legs, trunk, and neck. People with ALS lose the ability to move their limbs or to breathe independently. Owen is married with 3 children, though he lives in another state with the support of family members other than his wife and children. Owen's story describes how a catastrophic disability has affected his work and life as he ages.

I was introduced to computers while stationed in Germany by an officer who just bought a PC. He taught me the basics. I immediately applied it to the Army computer that handled all the maintenance records in our repair shop. I was the officer in charge of a 150-man company whose mission was to repair equipment for our customers who owned tents to tanks! After the Army, I was hired because of my experience with computers by the Department of Defense. I loved that project because I worked with soldiers again. As I learned more about how to operate computers, I would teach others what to do to get better results. I love teaching!

After the D.O.D. job, we moved to Memphis for another job in computer software development. I was a manager of 14 business systems advisors who wrote computer software specifications for the [company's] internal customers. My team wrote the specs for the mechanical maintenance of the airplanes. Our customers were the people who routed each jet to their next airport for repair. It was a brilliant design because they knew where certain mechanics could do the repairs.

I have 22 years of experience with developing software for computers. I wanted to become a teacher, but my dad said teaching was a dead end job and you don't make any money. I was young and believed my father, but to this day I wish that I became a teacher.

I got my ALS diagnosis in January 2005 and worked until June 2006. At first, I wore a knee brace because of my left leg was weak, then came my cane. The really tough part was telling my management and employees that I could not continue to be a manager. At one point, a female employee started to cry, and then I followed with crying. I started using a walker, followed by a power wheelchair. I bought a van with a ramp so I could drive to work. I stepped down as a manager after I groomed my replacement.

The United States has a confusing mix of coverage for disabilities, health care, and aging. There are social health insurance programs at national and state government levels, a military service-related system, and private pay health care systems. The Americans with Disabilities Act, mentioned previously, protects the right to work, preventing discrimination against qualified people with disabilities in the private sector, and in state and local governments (Americans with Disabilities Act, 1990). At this point in his life, Owen is not employed. Based on his diagnosis, Owen receives health coverage as a former military serviceman. Also, ALS is on the list of conditions that automatically qualifies Owen for "presumptive disability" payments under Supplemental Security Disability Income (SSDI), part of the social health care system in the United States. The only therapies for ALS covered by insurance are the "make-him-comfortable" variety, his sister relates. Insurance does not cover new treatments or assistive technology communication devices for him. He pays those expenses out of pocket.

I hire college students and it's awesome because they really care for me, and they get tremendous experience in caring for a person with ALS! Through the years of hiring people, I know which people I feel comfortable with, usually within the first few minutes of the interview. [My sister] says I have a natural talent for reading people. My current team is awesome. I spend most of my day writing emails, texts, and daily reports for my caregivers on what to do under certain circumstances. Because I can't talk, it's important that [they] know exactly why I need certain things done correctly.

So you might be asking, how did I type this document? I have a special computer with a camera pointing at my eye. Through incredible advanced technology, the camera tracks the movement of my eye, and on my computer screen, wherever I look the mouse pointer follows. Then if I keep staring at the object, like a letter on an online keyboard, I can type letters. I can even surf the Internet and check my email. I do Facebook each day. I am the assistant web master for my Boy Scout troop.

Though his illness required Owen to move cross-country, away from his wife and children, he describes the decision as "living with ALS instead of dying with it." Owen requires 24-hour care for his personal needs. He is the manager for his caregiver support staff. He is now the teacher he never thought he would be, training caregivers and enabling them to train newcomers. Although the illness is life threatening, Owen sees health and purpose in his daily life. His story illustrates adaptation to a catastrophic illness.

SENSORY DISABILITY—UNITED KINGDOM

Sensory loss is a major cause of disability with advancing age. Low vision is in the top three most prevalent disabilities in older people (World Health Organization, 2011). Work tasks such as reading the mail and printed documents, writing, keyboarding, viewing the computer screen, and using machinery can be challenging. Most people develop low vision because of eye diseases and health conditions such as macular degeneration, cataract, glaucoma, and diabetes. While vision that is lost usually cannot be restored, many people can make the most of the vision they have and continue employment. Frank is an example of someone with a visual impairment who has recently changed his career path:

Frank, age 62, has been self-employed for the last 2½ years after deciding to take early retirement from teaching. He now works as an education advisor and also runs a catering business.

Frank offers advice and consultancy to parents of visually impaired children regarding education, and gives talks at parent support group meetings and schools.

A year ago, Frank decided to venture into new territory by setting up a catering business. Having worked as a public relations officer, career coordinator, and head of an English department, Frank was already equipped with leadership skills and management experience, in addition to possessing excellent communication skills. Frank advised:

"Consulting a friend who had been running her own catering business for 10 years also really helped me, as it gave me an insight into what is really involved in running a business of this nature. I think it is really important to do thorough research on running a business and go into it with your eyes open."

As part of his catering business, Frank deals with the marketing, sales, and administrative side of the business by taking the bookings and visiting potential clients and venues. His catering manager is responsible for the actual preparation and presentation of the food.

Frank uses a Braille notetaker for administrative tasks, and employs an aide to assist him when traveling to see clients. Accurately judging the size of venues can be problematic. Frank's philosophy is: "If you expect problems and try to find solutions, most of the issues that you may come across can be easily resolved." (Royal National Institute of Blind People [RNIB], 2012)

Assessment and provision of the correct equipment, along with training in use of the equipment, can assist people with a visual impairment to remain in work. Some reasonable adjustments that could be expected to be made in the workplace are as follows (RNIB, 2013):

- Providing equipment, such as a CCTV, or in Frank's case, a Braille notetaker

- Providing software, such as ZoomText (Ai Squared)/JAWS (Freedom Scientific)/Supernova (Dolphin)

- Changing the working environment, such as altering lighting levels

- Changing procedures (medical appointments about someone's disability are recorded as "disability-related leave" rather than sick leave) or enabling an employee to bring her service dog to the workplace (there may be some limitations [e.g., in a hospital to comply with infection control requirements])

- Making changes to a job description to reassign some duties to other staff

- Providing a support worker

Frank is an example of someone with a rich employment history who is now using his previous skills to develop his own business, aided by both equipment and an aide.

COGNITIVE AND EMOTIONAL CHANGES—UNITED STATES

Mental health problems are not a normal part of aging. Cognitive and emotional changes can encompass a number of conditions, but for the purposes of this chapter, Alzheimer's disease and depression will be discussed.

Alzheimer's disease is a condition that is affecting work performance in the aging population. It is the most common form of dementia, a general term for memory loss and other intellectual disabilities serious enough to interfere with daily life, including tasks at work. Alzheimer's disease accounts for 50% to 80% of people diagnosed with dementia. Alzheimer's disease is progressive, meaning symptoms gradually worsen over a number of years. Alzheimer's is the 6th leading cause of death in the United States (Alzheimer's Association, 2014). The disease impairs memory and learning, often manifesting as forgetting conversations, work requests, what transpired at a meeting, phone messages, or directions. However, memory for meaningful past activities will remain intact in the early stages. Individuals may become lost when walking in a large building or going to work, and may have difficulty carrying out tasks in the correct sequence. Making things or putting things together may become hard, even for handy or crafty people. Drawing (especially copying) becomes difficult. Employers and coworkers may notice changes in memory, initiation, increased time needed to complete tasks, and that tasks are unsatisfactorily performed or left undone (Öhman, Nygård, & Borell, 2001). The impact of the onset of dementia on work is illustrated by the experience of Rudy Rice, age 73, who was interviewed for the Daily Inter Lake in Montana.

> *Mr. Rice remembers many things about growing up with nine sisters on a farm on Whitefish Stage Road in Montana. "I've lost a whole bunch of memory," Mr. Rice said. "I graduated from Whitefish High School in 1957. After about a year, I went into the Army. Then Dad got sick and they gave me 'early out.'" A few years later, Mr. Rice went to work as a general laborer on a highway project. He learned how to run a road grader while on the job, and that become his career. His daughter noticed memory problems around 1997, when he was still driving a grader for a living. At that time, Mr. Rice was 58 years old. He said he was able to work for a few more years despite his growing memory problems because his job was repetitive, driving back and forth over sections of road. He remembers that his mother had similar problems. "Mom was a lot like me," he said. "She lost her bearings." He recalled that his mother liked to go to the grocery store, but she would get lost, just as he would now, trying to go on his own.* (Chase, n.d.)

Mr. Rice is an example of how repetition in task performance may prolong work for a person who has dementia. Problem solving aspects of a job that a worker may still perform could prolong work, resulting in better economic and psychological well-being for the worker, especially as the necessity for health insurance increases. The Americans with Disabilities Act (ADA, 1990) states that the workplace must provide reasonable accommodations for those with disabilities, including dementias (Sachs & Redd, 1993):

- If an individual is unable to perform the job but is otherwise qualified, the employer must modify the job to enable the person to work (unless employer can prove that doing so would pose an undue hardship on the business)

- Individuals must raise the issue of need for accommodation, otherwise the employer is not obligated to make accommodations

Evidence suggests that up to 25% of people over the age of 65 have symptoms of depression that are severe enough to require treatment (Williamson, 2012). Older people with physical illnesses are at increased risk of depression. Depression may lead to profound lifestyle, physical, economic, and psychological stresses on individuals and their families. Like any condition, depression may affect work abilities. Signs of depression at work may include disregard for personal hygiene, lack of engagement with coworkers, disinterest in work, fatigue, irritability, and calling in sick due to aches, pains, and digestive problems (Centers for Disease Control and Prevention, 2011). Older workers need to know that depression can be treated with antidepressants, psychosocial interventions such as cognitive behavioral therapy, or a mixture of both (Centers for Disease Control, 2011; National Institute for Health and Clinical Excellence, 2009). In 2007, the Sainsbury Centre for Mental Health provided a review of evidence to support keeping working age people healthy and promoting health in the workplace. Recommendations included promoting a culture of health in the workplace, such as openness about mental illness, and through this reducing stigma and encouraging help-seeking behavior. It recommended that companies should have health and well-being policies and improved access to psychological interventions in the workplace. In addition, employees should be aware of how to respond appropriately to colleagues who are showing signs of distress and withdrawal (Sainsbury Centre for Mental Health, 2007). The older worker should be made aware of these policies because stigma might prevent seeking support within the workplace. Individuals may be concerned about discrimination on the grounds of not only their mental health, but their age.

THE OLDER WORKING CAREGIVER—UNITED KINGDOM

Gian is a surgeon of international reputation. At age 93, he is a man of great dignity and privacy. With an economy of carefully selected words, Gian relates his wife's long slide into dementia and its impact on their lives. Camilla's dementia began when she and Gian were both middle-aged. Their two children were grown and gone. Gian was at the peak of his career as a surgeon and medical professor at a nearby university in the United Kingdom. Gian's story relates the influence of the illness of another person on his aging, work, and life.

> *Camilla died by degrees. Eventually, she could recognize no one; not me, not our own children. When she was young, we frequently entertained at home. We traveled around the world when I had speaking engagements. As her dementia progressed, we could not even get across London. The stations are poorly accessible to people with disabilities.*
>
> *When Camilla's illness worsened, it seemed as though it took weeks for someone to fit the need. I was told to put her in a care home, but I could not. This is the only home she needed. Eventually, I hired nurses to care for her around the clock. As I lost more and more of her, I became single, but not single. I could ask a woman to accompany me to a dinner or a meeting once, but not again. It was not proper.*

The UK National Health Service provided benefits, but they were unsatisfactory for Gian's expectations for his wife. Financially, Gian was able to pay for private care, but it meant that he must continue to work until a late age. Instead of retiring to enjoy a life of leisure, he continued a rigorous schedule. At about age 70, he recounts, he had to discontinue performing surgery because a tremor developed in his dominant hand. When pressed, he did say that he mourned the loss of the use of his hands for surgery as an "irreplaceable art." He remained at the University, teaching medical students and residents. Eventually, his travels were severely curtailed by back pain and subsequent laminectomy. Gian discounts his own experience with disability and aging, relating it as overshadowed by his wife's illness. He describes losing her in little bits and pieces as agonizing. Camilla finally died after 30 years of dementia, when Gian was 83. She was 79.

> *I have lived a long and full life. My work is nearly finished. If you want to come back to see me, I suggest you do it soon.*

With the support of a secretary, Gian continues a regular workweek to catalog his books, journals, and papers, packaging them for shipment to public and private libraries around the world. He is still asked to lecture and travel, but has curtailed these activities because his endurance is failing.

LABOR FORCE DYNAMICS

The U.S. Department of Health and Human Services (USDHHS) reports in its publication *Growing Older in America: The Health and Retirement Study,* that 35% of respondents age 55 to 59 cited poor health as being "very important" in their decision to retire (USDHHS, n.d.). Salm reports that declining health has also been found to be a reason for involuntary job loss (2009). Older people with and without disabilities have "pull" factors to continue working, and "push" factors to retire. Neither circumstance is free from pressures or inducements. Push and pull factors include financial stability, staying healthy and active, work environment, family responsibilities, status, and social contact. A person's sense of self-determination at work and the degree to which the workplace "fits" also contributes to the push and pull for aging workers with disabilities. Some older workers will move to self-employment as an alternative, some by preference and others by poor job prospects, poor job fit, or low salary (Zissimopoulous & Karoly, 2009). De Lange, Schalk, and van der Heijden describe additional factors that make it difficult for people to remain in the workplace, both individual and environmental (2013). Workforce participation rates of older people vary widely, depending on many personal and environmental factors. The most common personal factors affecting work include health issues, changing priorities, life role transitions, economic status, age, and particular traits such as self-esteem and attitudes toward work (Schalk et al., 2010). Environmental influences include events in the immediate community and in the larger world. They include social networks, corporate restructuring, political and economic upheaval, legislation, and human resource policy changes. Each person has a unique view of work, preference for contributing, and set of living circumstances. Some higher income workers engaged in physically demanding and mentally taxing activities may choose different work, or may retire at a younger age. Jannetje and her husband moved from an urban to a rural setting. Their work and method of productivity changed from employee to self-employed, a style that enabled them to have maximum flexibility and personal satisfaction. People who live active lives in middle age are more likely to be active as elders, regardless of whether they have a disability, but conditions that routinely occur as part of the natural aging process may impact the ability to work (Caban-Martinez et al., 2011; von Bonsdorff et al., 2011). For example, approximately half of adults over age 65 in the United States have some arthritis-related condition (Centers for Disease Control and Prevention, 2011). Arthritis is indiscriminate, affecting all social classes and types of workers in all countries. Jannetje, Owen, Gian, and many others share the impact of long-term conditions on their completion of daily tasks.

Economics have a large influence on work and retirement. Lower income workers are more impacted by physical disabilities. They may experience a loss of productivity as their health deteriorates, and work longer hours to meet their financial needs. Earnings for older workers may not stretch quite as far to cover age-related increases in health insurance costs or private, out-of-pocket costs for those with national health plans. They may be caught in a downward economic spiral, having to work past a preferred retirement age just to make ends meet. A growing percentage of older people will continue to work out of financial necessity (Caban-Martinez et al., 2011). Though in a higher income category, Gian continued to be productive late in life for financial reasons and by personal preference. He continued his work to cover extraordinary expenses for Camilla and for the sense of community denied him by the loss of his partner to dementia. Some older people continue to work as a result of financial necessity, some by preference, and some by workforce demand. There may not be younger workers available to fill the widespread needs of the community (Purcell, 2009). Healthcare workers retire at younger ages than workers in other professions, thus decreasing the number of providers available to care for an increasing number of older people. Moranda (2011) suggests that nurses, in particular, may "age out" of physically demanding jobs to retire at an age well below the statistical average.

OCCUPATIONAL ADAPTATION

Society cannot assume any common pattern of aging, disability, or employment needs. Some people have the desire to work, but cannot because of individual or environmental factors. None of the people who told their stories for this chapter described an experience of employment discrimination on the basis of age or disability; however, it continues to occur. Explicit and implicit bias persists in the workplace, regardless of legislation. There is a cultural bias that older workers appear disabled, whether or not they are qualified for the job and able to perform. The bias is greater for adults over 50 years of age, regardless of ability (Draper, Reid, & McMahon, 2012). In times of economic uncertainty, workers over 50 who may have held their positions for many years are subject to downsizing, layoffs, and loss of health benefits. Sipprelle and Newman interviewed 100 Americans over 50, some with identified disabilities and some without, who thought they were "set for life," yet lost their jobs in the recent recession (2012). Many interviewees in the *Over 50 and Out of Work* project describe desperation with age-related changes in health, the high cost or loss of health insurance, and the desire to work but inability to find employment (Sipprelle & Newman, 2012).

Some people growing older with an identified disability, like Jannetje, may continue to be active and participate fully in their communities. She remains productive with limited modifications and no governmental benefits. Other people may be considered "fit to work," but may lack the support necessary to do so. Yet others receiving disability benefits, such as Owen, would be better described as prematurely retired. Owen's dramatic loss of physical abilities in middle age overwhelmed his ability to continue in his same work role, changing his routines and social identity. For him, disability brought fear, frustration, and guilt as his ability to be productive changed. He has found creative ways to continue productive roles as a husband, a parent, a friend, a teacher, and a community member.

Each of those interviewed for this chapter faced challenges in his or her adjustment to aging, disability, and work. One perspective relevant to this process is Schkade and Schultz's theoretical model of occupational adaptation (1992). This model outlines the process by which a person makes sense of and interacts with his or her environment. The theoretical model postulates that as an individual adapts, his or her function subsequently increases. Responding to life challenges is referred to as *occupational adaptation*. The interviewees perceived environmental work demands, to which they responded with unique adaptive strategies. As Jannetje ages, she uses strategies that she established early in life and practiced across time to retain her role as an independent worker. She uses her adaptive capacity to alter the strategies as her needs change. For Owen, the mismatch between environmental demands, his physical ability, and his desire to work created a precipitous need to change. Owen's adaptive capacity was stretched to the limit as he lost mobility, verbal communication, and independence. Owen used a great deal of effort—of adaptive energy—to change, brought about by an inevitable imbalance with work and life. Frank found a new work role and made adaptations to succeed in this role through assistive technology, in the form of a notetaker and an aide.

PERSPECTIVES FROM ACROSS THE GLOBE

Health issues inevitably increase as we grow older, but aging is not synonymous with disability, nor is disability synonymous with ill health. Several centers are involved in clarifying and forming solutions for the issues of aging, disability, and work. The Sloan Center on Aging & Work at Boston College has invited international researchers to study topics on aging in the workplace. The National Technical Assistance and Research Leadership Center has produced websites, briefs, papers, reports, podcasts, and webinars addressing workforce issues for adults with disabilities.

Heidkamp et al. (2012) and Johnson (2011) of the National Technical Assistance and Research Leadership Center have written extensively regarding disability issues and policies, posing specific solutions. The World Health Organization (WHO) *International Classification of Functioning, Disability and Health* document, known as the ICF, includes worldwide individual and societal perspectives on disability, activity, and participation (WHO, 2014). The WHO perceives changes in health to be a universal human experience. The ICF acknowledges that every human being may experience a decrease in health sometime in life, with a subsequent loss of ability based on cultural, social, and environmental contributors to a person's quality of life. The ICF illustrates a continuum of health and ability, including cultural assumptions regarding the impact of disability and aging influence policies and program development. Further, the WHO and the World Bank Group jointly produced the *World Report on Disability* (2014) to provide ideas for innovative policies and programs, with the intent of improving the quality of life for people with disabilities. This report contains information to help the reader understand and measure disability, health, rehabilitation, assistance and support, enabling environments, education, and employment.

Considerations for the Future

An aging society brings unprecedented demands on health care systems, support services, public accommodation, and strategies for employment. Morris advocates for changes in disability welfare, seeking reasonable adjustments and decreasing prejudices with a wide perspective (2011). She suggests the discussion is no longer about disability rights, but about larger issues of sustainability, underlying causes of inequality, and political and economic concerns. Too many systems suffer from disjointed requirements and poor communication. Systems vary according to the degree of government involvement and the culture unique to each country. Governments face difficult choices to balance the budgets and provide services for their citizens. Forming reasonable solutions requires careful, accurate needs assessment and coordination of individuals, services, and communities to design dynamic solutions.

Heidkamp, Mabe, and DeGraaf (2012) describe recommendations to expand existing services in the United States, including older worker task forces, employer outreach and education programs, one-stop career centers, and workforce development initiatives. Facilitating partnerships and communication within and amongst organizations decreases duplication and red tape. Recommended changes focus on policy and legislation, technical assistance and training, and research. Goals for policy changes include changes to public pension eligibility, and updated age discrimination legislation. Related goals for technical assistance and training include access to degrees and certification, lifelong learning opportunities, affordable modifications universal to all workers, and education in digital literacy that leads to employment in high-demand, high-wage fields. Training seminars and workshops for coaches and workforce developers will share effective strategies across aging, disability, and employment needs. Expending resources to implement technical assistance and training will support economic security for individuals and communities.

The recommended changes described will result in alterations to the culture of communities and countries. Gustafsson, Andersson, Andersson, Fjellstro, and Sidenvall (2003) recognize that old age and changing abilities of workers threaten established, culturally defined values. New programs creating a culture of support for older workers, making use of their expertise, exploring flexible patterns of work, and modifying worker supports or assistance programs may also threaten culturally defined values. A changing culture may serve to decrease the stigma attached to the labels of "disabled" and "old." New legislation in Australia is groundbreaking in the area of alternatives to traditional retirement. Caban-Martinez et al. (2011) describe a culture of support that includes coordinated, comprehensive health and disability insurance to address the needs of elder workers. Cooke (2006) describes the Workforce Aging in the New Economy (WANE) project in Canada, including how new pathways to flexible and phased retirement will keep talent in the workplace. Complex human capital strategies will be needed to fully consider the needs of older workers with disabilities.

Conclusion

This chapter examined concepts related to people aging with a lifelong disability, people acquiring a disability as they age, the impact of being a caregiver for someone with a disability, and the influence of this on their lives and work. The people interviewed in this chapter have widely different disabilities, and work and life experiences. As our lives and our activities change, our very definition of work also changes. Each person interviewed for this chapter is aging with a disability that reveals different needs, adaptive strategies, and perspectives on work. Jannetje, Owen, and Gian each commented on the use of their hands as integral to their work. As their abilities have changed, each described their work as becoming more than gainful employment. For them, work is about participating, contributing, and living a productive life of the mind and heart. They describe an engagement of the self—using one's talents and gifts as part of a community—despite the influences of age and disability. As people live longer lives and abilities change, lifework is a valuable concept, worthy of additional consideration in the definition of activity and participation. As Jannetje most eloquently says, "Your work changes and so do you. Nothing stays the same." Clearly, there is no single solution to the issue of aging, disability, and work. Society needs to search for excellent solutions instead of perfect ones. Society needs to consider the idea of universal opportunity, a concept that changes as people and environments change.

References

Alzheimer's Association. (2014). *2014 Alzheimer's Disease Facts and Figures.* Retrieved May 21, 2014 from http://www.alz.org/downloads/Facts_Figures_2014.pdf.

Americans With Disabilities Act 1990, Amended. Pub. L. No. 110-325, Title 42, § 12102 [Section 3] (2009). Retrieved June 26, 2013 from http://www.ada.gov/pubs/adastatute08.htm#12102.

Australian Bureau of Statistics. (2010). Older people and the labour market. *Australian Social Trends.* cat. no. 4102.0 Retrieved June 26, 2013 from http://www.abs.gov.au/AUSSTATS/abs@.nsf/Lookup/4102.0Main+Features40March+Quarter+2012#end9.

Australian Government Department of Health. (2000). National Strategy for an Ageing Australia. Retrieved from http://www.health.gov.au/internet/main/publishing.nsf/Content/health-budget2000-fact-acfact1.htm.

Australian Government Department of Human Services. (2012). Retrieved from http://www.humanservices.gov.au/customer/services/medicare/medicare?utm_id=9#N1006D.

Australian Institute of Health and Welfare. (2008). Retrieved June 26, 2013, from http://www.aihw.gov.au/definition-of-disability/.

Beecher, H. W. (1895) *The Teachers' Institute, 18*(1), 16.

Caban-Martinez, A.J., Lee, D.J., Fleming, L.E., Tancredi, D.J., Arheart, K.L., LeBlanc, W.F., . . . Meunnig, P.A. (2011). Arthritis, occupational class and the aging US workforce. *American Journal of Public Health, 101*(9), 1729-1734.

Carnoy, M. (2000). *Sustaining the new economy: Work, family, and community in the information age.* New York: Russell Sage Foundation.

Centers for Disease Control and Prevention. (August 1, 2011). Retrieved June 26, 2013, from http://www.cdc.gov/arthritis/data_statistics/arthritis_related_stats.htm#3.

Chase, C. (n.d.). Man, family walk to end Alzheimer's. *The Daily Inter Lake.* Retrieved from http://www.dailyinterlake.com/.

Cooke, M. (2006). Policy changes and the labour force participation of older workers: Evidence from six countries. *Canadian Journal on Aging, 25*(4), 387-400.

De Lange, A. H., Schalk, R., & van der Heijden, B. I. J. M., (2013). Sustainable work functioning across the life span? (Ouder worden en duuzame inzetbarrheid op het werk?) In W.B. Schaufeli, & A. Bakker (Eds.), *The psychology of work and health* (pp. 381-398). Houten: Bohn stafleu van Loghum.

Draper, W. R., Reid, C. A., & McMahon, B. T. (2012). Workplace discrimination and the perception of disability. *Rehabilitation Counseling Bulletin, 55,* 29-37.

Equality Act. (2010). London; Stationery Office. Retrieved June 26, 2013, from http://www.legislation.gov.uk/ukpga/2010/15/section/6.

Gustafsson, K., Andersson, I., Andersson, J., Fjellstro, C., & Sidenvall, B. (2003). Older women's perceptions of independence versus dependence in food-related work. *Public Health Nursing, 20,* 237-247.

Haight, J. M. (2003). Human error and the challenges of an aging workforce. *Professional Safety, 48*(12), 1-9.

Heidkamp, M., Mabe, W., & DeGraaf, B. (2012). The public workforce system: Serving older job seekers and the disability implications of an aging workforce. *Report NTAR Leadership Center.* New Brunswick, NJ: John J. Heldrich Center for Workforce Development, Rutgers University.

Jeszeck, C., DeFrank, T, Leavitt, K., Peterson, J.S., Peterson, J., Tai, Y., & Wial, H. (2007.) International responses to an aging labor force: Lessons for U.S. policy. In T. Ghilarducci & J. Turner. (Eds.), *Work options for older Americans* (pp. 321-346). Notre Dame, IN: University of Notre Dame Press.

Johnson, R. W. (2011). Impact of federal policies on an aging workforce with disabilities. *Report NTAR Leadership Center.* New Brunswick, NJ: John J. Heldrich Center for Workforce Development, Rutgers University.

McFarlin, D. B., Song, J., & Sonntag, M. (1991). Integrating the disabled into the workforce: A survey of Fortune-500 company attitudes and practices. *Employee Responsibility and Rights Journal, 4,* 107-123.

McMullin, J., & Shuey, K. M. (2006). Ageing, disability and workplace accommodations. *Ageing and Society, 26,* 831-847.

Moranda, C. (2011). Return to work: Addressing the "aging out" problem in the workplace. *Professional Case Management, 16,* 218-220.

Morris, J. (2011). *Rethinking disability policy.* York: Joseph Rowntree Foundation. Retrieved June 26, 2013, from http://www.jrf.org.uk/publications/rethinking-disability-policy.

National Disability Insurance Scheme. (2012). Retrieved February 8, 2013, from http://www.ndis.gov.au/.

National Institute for Health and Clinical Excellence. (2009). *Depression in adults (update) (CG90).* Retrieved June 26, 2013, from http://www.nice.org.uk/CG90.

Öhman, A., Nygård, L., & Borell, L. (2001). The vocational situation in cases of memory deficits or younger-onset dementia. *Scandinavian Journal of Caring Sciences, 15,* 34-43.

Purcell, P. J. (2009). Older workers: Employment and retirement trends. *Journal of Deferred Compensation, 14*(2), 85-104.

Royal National Institute of Blind People. (2013). Frank's Story. Retrieved June 25, 2014, from http://www.rnib.org.uk/information-everyday-living-work-and-employment-success-stories/franks-story.

Sachs, P. R., & Redd, C. A. (1993). The Americans with Disabilities Act and individuals with neurological impairments. *Rehabilitation Psychology, 38*(2), 87-101.

Sainsbury Centre for Mental Health. (2007). *Call for evidence by the National Director for Health and Work. How can we keep working age people healthy and how can the workplace be used to promote health?* Retrieved June 27, 2013, from http://www.centreformentalhealth.org.uk/pdfs/scmh_health_work_wellbeing_evidence.pdf.

Salm, M. (2009). Does job loss cause ill health? [Abstract]. *Health Economics, 18,* 1075-1089.

Schalk, R., van Veldhoven, M., de Lange, A. H., De Witte, H., Kraus, K., Stamov-Roßnagel, C., . . . Zacher, H. (2010). Moving European research on work and ageing forward: Overview and agenda. *European Journal of Work and Organizational Psychology, 19,* 76-101.

Schkade, J., & Schultz, S. (1992). Occupational adaptation: Toward a holistic approach for contemporary practice, part 1. *American Journal of Occupational Therapy, 46,* 829-837.

Sipprelle, S. M., & Newman, S. D., (2012). *Over 50 and out of work.* Retrieved June 20, 2013, from http://www.overfiftyandoutofwork.com/.

Stock, W. A., & Beegle, K. (2004). Employment protections for older workers: Do disability discrimination laws matter? *Contemporary Economic Policy, 22,* 111-126.

Toossi, M. (2007). Employment outlook: 2006–16: Labor force projections to 2016: More workers in their golden years. *Monday Labor Review, 130*(11), 33-52.

Turner, J. A. (2008). Work options for older Americans: Employee benefits for the era of living longer. *Benefits Quarterly, 24,* 20-25.

United Nations. (2006). *Convention on the Rights of Persons with Disabilities, Article 1.* Retrieved from http://www.un.org/disabilities/default.asp?id=261.

U.S. Department of Health and Human Services. *Growing older in America: The health and retirement study.* Ann Arbor, MI: University of Michigan. Retrieved from http://hrsonline.isr.umich.edu/sitedocs/databook/HRS_Text_WEB_ch2.pdf.

U.S. Equal Employment Opportunity Commission. (1967). The Age Discrimination and Employment Act of 1967. Retrieved June 24, 2014, from http://www.eeoc.gov/laws/statutes/adea.cfm.

von Bonsdorff, M.B., Seitsamo, J., Ilmarinen, J., Nygård, C-H., von Bonsdorff, M.E., Rantanen, T. (2011). Work ability in midlife as a predictor of mortality and disability in later life: A 28-year prospective follow-up study. *Canadian Medical Association Journal, 183*(4), E235-E242.

Williamson, T. (2012). *Mental health and later life.* Mental Health Foundation. Retrieved, June 26, 2013, from http://www.mentalhealth.org.uk/our-news/blog/12-03-26/.

World Health Organization. (2014). International Classification of Functioning Disability and Health (ICF). Retrieved from http://www.who.int/classifications/icf/en/.

Zissimopoulos, J. M., & Karoly, L. A. (2009). Labor-force dynamics at older ages: Movements into self-employment for workers and nonworkers. *Research on Aging, 31*(1), 89-111.

6

Well-Being and Employment

Linda A. Hunt, PhD, OTR/L, FAOTA

Work to me is a sacred thing.—Margaret Bourke-White (1963)

The culture of retirement is changing. Baby Boomers continue to work past retirement age for sustained financial security. Others are working because they simply enjoy it. Still, some older adults may work because it provides role identity, purpose, being with others, and continuity in lifestyle. Evidence is building that continued employment in the right environment may contribute to better quality of life and longevity. In future years, this trend of delayed retirement may continue as work becomes less physically demanding due to technology innovations, such as the use of robots performing heavy lifting, fine motor coordination demands, and repetitive aspects of some labor and manufacturing jobs. Another current trend is making a gradual transition from full-time employment to full-time retirement by having a *bridge job* (Pitt-Catsouphes & Smyer, 2006). By working part-time, older people are able to engage in activities outside of work that prior time restraints did not allow.

Having the option to continue to participate in the labor force can have important positive health consequences for older workers. "Quality" jobs may benefit employees' physical and mental health, making it less likely that they will experience certain conditions that can accelerate the aging process. The Committee for Economic Development Studies (1999) found a positive relationship between employment and physical and mental well-being. A recent study showed that the mental health status of employed older workers is better than for those in full-time retirement (James, Besen, Matz-Costa, & Pitt-Catsouphes, 2010). In another study, nearly half of respondents said that their desire to keep active was also an important factor in the decisions they made with regard to work and retirement (Moen, Erickson, Argarwal, Fields, & Todd, 2000).

Rowe and Kahn (1997) defined successful aging as multidimensional, encompassing the avoidance of disease and disability, the maintenance of high physical and cognitive function, and sustained engagement in social and productive activities. They defined productive activities as

Hunt LA, Wolverson C.
Work and the Older Person: Increasing Longevity and Well-Being (pp 63-73).
© 2015 SLACK Incorporated.

working, volunteering, or caregiving. More recently, Robert Hormats (2012), U.S. Under Secretary of State for Economic Growth, Energy, and the Environment, confirmed this, "We need a sea change not just in policies, but in attitudes about what it means to grow old. We must break the stereotype that to be old is to be inactive or dependent, and in so doing turn 'population aging' into the century's greatest achievement" (2012). Hormats was sworn into his government position at age 66. Butler (1975) was one of the first advocates of older people and recognized that age is incorrectly associated with diminished capabilities and dwindling contributions. These inaccurate perceptions are detrimental to both older people and the broader society. Furthermore, Rowe and Kahn (1997) highlighted education as a major determinant of occupation and the ability to remain working into old age. The Baby Boomer generation has the highest percentage of college graduates in comparison to previous cohorts going through the aging process. Those with greater formal education seem to stay employed as they age.

Work serves as a source of identity and resources. A recent study confirms that retiring before age 62 years can be detrimental for both subjective physical and emotional health. Data were taken from the Health and Retirement Study, a nationally representative, biennial panel survey of older Americans and their spouses. This study began in 1992 and has data available through 2008 (University of Michigan, 2012). Researchers selected their sample from the 9,753 individuals, born between 1931 and 1941, that became Health and Retirement Study cohort respondents in 1992. Given the interest in the effects of the transition from the labor force into retirement, they used a labor force status variable (combining information from self-reported retirement status, working for pay, hours of work, and several other indicators) to omit 1,640 individuals who were partly or fully retired at the first wave, and 1,489 individuals who were out of the labor force for reasons other than retirement at all observed time points, or at least at all the observed time points prior to their retirement (if they retired). The resulting sample included 6,624 individuals. Excluded were all preretirement records when a respondent was not in the labor force currently, as well as those records when a respondent reported being retired currently but was out of the labor force at the wave directly preceding retirement. As a result, researchers used 56,796 records in the analyses. Only 210 individuals died before their transition to retirement; thus, mortality is unlikely to introduce a substantial selection bias into the study's results. Selection bias was also minimized because the sample included those 333 individuals who were still not retired and remained in the labor force in 2010.

Data were based on self-reports of health and depressive symptoms. Assessing depressive symptoms included use of the Center for Epidemiologic Studies Depression scale, which asks: "Now think about the week and the feelings you have experienced. Please tell me if each of the following was true for you much of the time this past week: you were happy; you enjoyed life; you felt lonely; you felt depressed; you felt sad; you could not get going; you felt that everything you did was an effort; your sleep was restless." The study concluded that retiring prior to age 62 can be problematic for both subjective physical and emotional health. They did not find any pronounced disadvantages associated with late retirement (Calvo, Sarkisian, & Tamborinai, 2013).

An engaged and purposeful lifestyle brings a wide range of benefits, including increased longevity, resistance to dementia, and enhanced cognitive flexibility (Stine-Morrow, Parisi, Morrow, & Park, 2008). This chapter focuses on how employment, an example of an engaged and purposeful lifestyle, may also contribute to longevity. Research mostly focuses on characteristics found in purposeful engagement, which is characteristic of employment. Therefore, the chapter discusses and relies on research outcomes from studies examining engagement in purposeful activities, empowerment, socialization, physical and emotional well-being, and economic well-being to argue that staying employed—in some capacity that is favorable to the person—is beneficial for the individual and society as a whole. Through case studies and narratives, this chapter illustrates and substantiates that work contributes to longevity. The following is an interview with Eileen Jones, who lives in Montana. At age 97, she is one of the oldest workers in the United States. The interview highlights many points made in this chapter about work and successful aging.

At what age did you retire?

I retired at 62. Then at 88, I received a phone call from a woman who asked me if I wanted to work part-time for the Office of Public Assistance. The job was actually for the Experience Works Program. This program recruits older adults. It helps people learn the skills for a job at a particular place of employment. Then when they have learned the skills, they apply for the job. I have worked here for 9 years. They call me "jack of all trades" because I do a little of everything. I file papers, wait on customers when they walk in the door, answer the phone, put application packets together, and I take care of the incoming and outgoing mail. I work 20 hours a week and divide it up into 3 days.

Have you worked all your life?

Yes, I am from the old school. I have always showed up on time, did the job I was supposed to do, and only took off for vacations. I worked while I lived with my parents and paid them rent from my earnings to help them out. We were poor. I did go to a 2-year college.

What do you like about working?

It gets me out of the apartment. It keeps me social. I like to be with people, to meet new people. I have a good sense of humor and I can only use it when I am around people. Those I work with like my sense of humor. People are kind to me at work. They take me as I am. They call me the "big boss." They tell me I brighten the office. I tease the caseworkers and they love it. I do not feel lonely when I am at work. Also, it helps me financially.

Do you have any final comments for me about working as an older person?

Working gives me purpose. It is good for the mind. I can still do math in my head. It may not be for everyone because as we get older, some people get sick. I am lucky. I only use a cane once in awhile. I still drive.

You are remarkable.

Yes I am! God is good to me.

ENGAGEMENT IN PURPOSEFUL ACTIVITIES

A report from the American Association of Retired Persons (AARP, 2003) found older workers today look to and expect dynamic retirements. They want stimulating environments where they have plenty of choices to engage in meaningful activities. Although most who are approaching retirement envision their retirement as a period that will include leisurely pursuits, new experiences, and time spent with loved ones, the majority also expect their retirement to include some form of work and purpose for how they spend the rest of their lives. Older workers who find that their employment creates opportunities to contribute to others find that they are also contributing to their own well-being. Gruenewald, Liao, and Seeman (2013) found that feeling needed and useful may be linked to health trajectories in later life. Not feeling needed by others predicted greater risk of institutionalization and death. Those who feel that they are needed and useful to others may take better care of themselves to maintain their ability to contribute, engage in more social and productive activity, and experience greater affective well-being, all of which may be paths to better physical well-being. This is demonstrated by Philip Coster, age 66, of the Pacific Northwest.

Philip took an early retirement at age 54. He is a member of the Baby Boom generation, the first generation that talked about taking early retirement. He was tired of the 10-hour days and decided that he did not "need a ton of money." However, he went back to work, as he wanted to "stay in the game." He enjoys meeting new people, and his new job is a continuation of his career in sales. He reports that he does feel better working again because his job requires communication skills and the use of technology. He likes making connections that benefit people. When he cuts back on his employment hours, he will pick up volunteer activities. His next goals are to work with veterans who have disabilities. He wants to teach disabled veterans to play golf for better mental and physical well-being. He also has plans to mentor at-risk youth. Mr. Coster reflects that he is the beginning of the aging Baby Boomers. "We will define what it means to age, and while we are aging, give back." He believes that staying purposeful is the best way to age. He wants to take care of his health so that he can continue to contribute.

Professors in higher education exemplify this concept of feeling needed and useful to others in their desire to work beyond age 65. Mandatory retirement in higher education employment was eliminated on January 1, 1994. With this change, the United States became one of the few countries in the world to offer true lifetime employment security for tenured faculty members. The lifting of mandatory retirement occurred just as the wave of faculty hired in the early 1960s was about to reach traditional retirement age, prompting some critics to argue that the higher education system soon would be overwhelmed by a gerontacracy of aging teachers and scholars (Ashenfelter & Card, 2001). Some would argue that mandatory retirement would open up opportunities for younger people, who today spend as long as 10 to 12 years pursuing careers from which senior faculty members refuse to retire. Others believe that if professors initially hired in the 1960s, 1970s, or 1980s—a far more pedagogically diverse era than today—choose to remain on staff, then current students will benefit by having a few more years to sample courses in important subfields that soon will be redefined beyond recognition or will vanish from the curriculum entirely (Johnson, 2010). In *The Chronicle of Higher Education,* June (2012) reports that aging professors create a faculty bottleneck because 1 in 3 professors are age 60 or older at some universities, especially at the private universities, such as Cornell, Duke, George Mason, and Claremont McKenna College.

Aging professors have usually developed careers at a single institution, and often, the research they have created has built the reputation of that university. At some universities, the culture has provided built-in flexibility of hours and workloads in the right environment that supports older workers, a reason that many older workers stay employed. Aside from the usual perks of working, such as health insurance and good benefits, teaching at a university provides intellectual stimulation, camaraderie, access to cultural events, interaction with interesting people of various ages, and opportunities for travel. Most professors report that the job continues to maintain their identity and purpose, while contributing to society. Here are some quotes from older professors about engagement in purposeful work (June, 2012):

- "As long as I can do the job, I'm going to keep doing it." (Age 68)
- "If a person is still performing very well, I don't see why people should suggest that there's a moral or other obligation to let somebody else come in." (Age 68)
- "Everybody that knows me knows I'm going out of here feet first." (Age 68)
- "Right now I'm at a really exciting place in my research. I'd like to hang in there and see where it goes." (Age 81)
- "I have had so many students tell me that my course changed their life." (Age 73)
- "Despite mythology to the contrary, there's very little evidence that older faculty members become less productive. Faculty at top research universities, in particular, are more productive because tenure and rich resources work together in their favor." (Age 69)
- "That's why it's hard to think about retiring. I just keep thinking of things I want to do. My career is moving along, and it's more and more exciting. Why quit now?" (Age 68)
- "It's a very exciting course to teach. I hate to give it up by retiring." (Age 69)

All of these older professors talk about how vibrant and healthy they feel. They tie this vitality to their passion for their work and the purpose that it provides for them. They seem not to dwell on what they have done, but what they hope to accomplish in the future. Another theme that came through is that time has given them wisdom. When people feel that they can contribute their lifelong wisdom to others in a work setting, this motivates them to continue working. For example, Spencer Michels from PBS interviewed California Governor Jerry Brown (Michels, 2013). Mr. Michels asked Governor Brown how he was feeling since he was diagnosed with prostate cancer. The Governor responded that:

> At 75, it is not like being 55, much less 45. You get older. You can't run as fast, you have to watch your diet a little more. That is just the way it is. But I will tell you, in my life, I have been able to devote a lot of my time to studying California, to studying how its process of government works, and I really feel more equipped physically, intellectually, and spiritually to do this work than I ever have in any other time in my life.

In 2011, Bel Kaufman, at age 99, became the oldest known hired professor when she was hired by her alma mater Hunter College to teach as an adjunct professor on Jewish humor. During her first semester of instruction, she reported, "I'm too busy to get old." Kaufman still teaches and spends her days writing a book, *Dear Papa*, about her grandfather, the famous Sholem Aleichem, who wrote the stories that became *Fiddler on the Roof*. She was in her 50s when she wrote the famous novel, *Up the Down Staircase*. She now meets former students who are grandparents. In an interview published in *Vogue*, Kaufman told Robert Sullivan:

> I've lived a long time, a very long time, 101 years, and I'm still here. I'm done with the doubts and struggles and insecurities of youth. I'm finished with loss and guilt and regret. I'm very old, and nothing is expected of me. Now, provided good health continues, I can do what I want. I can write my memoirs. I can edit my works for future eBooks. I can even do nothing—what a luxury that is! I have new priorities and a new appreciation of time. I enjoy my family more than ever, and also a sunny day and a comfortable bed. I keep up my interest in books and theater and people, and when I'm tired, I rest. My former students write to me and visit me. I had many problems and disasters in my life; fortunately, at my age I don't remember what they were. I'm glad I am 101. (Sullivan, 2012)

EMPOWERMENT, WORK, AND HEALTH

At age 101, Bel Kaufman finds purpose in her work and also empowerment. She works on what she wants to do. Empowerment enables autonomy and control over one's work. People who are empowered at work use their skills and abilities to benefit both their organization and themselves. Empowerment of older people is a widely held goal among health care practitioners (Rowe & Kahn, 1997). Working in an environment that empowers individuals may serve to protect integrity, lucidity, and longevity, restoring for society an enormous resource in the experience and wisdom of its older members. Alexander, Langer, Newman, Chandler, and Davies (1989) wrote about empowerment from within through mindfulness practice and transcendental meditation. Having perceived control added to longevity. Older people who have mastered job skills over time may experience an inner empowerment that may bring job satisfaction to them and may also contribute to their ability to mentor others, which also contributes to job satisfaction (Wåhlin, Ek, & Idvall, 2010). Here is an example of an older worker teaching and mentoring a younger person, who now is empowered to possibly pass his craft on to another generation.

> Lee Miller, age 57, explained in an interview for the Wall Street Journal that he learned his trade at age 23 from legendary boot maker Charlie Dunn, who was 79 years old at the time. Dunn made boots until he was 88, and died at age 95. Miller states that he will continue to make boots as long as he can. Miller's mentor was empowered by his boot making ability, and this empowerment has transferred to Miller: "No automated machine can do work as fine as the human can." Miller continues to depend on aging boot makers to improve his skills. He seeks them out at boot making conventions, wanting to borrow and preserve their techniques. (Silverman, 2012)

Denmark and Williams talk about their experiences with aging in academia, and the empowerment of mentoring students and colleagues (2012). Denmark reports:

> *One of the high points in my career is when former students who are well established in their own careers, as well as people from abroad whom I've interacted with, tell me and others what a great mentor I have been and how important I have been in their profession.*

She continues to talk about the power of mentoring, which comes after one has worked in a field for a long time and has become recognized as an expert or authority in a particular field. Mentors are needed in all work settings. Older workers may feel invigorated and empowered as they guide emerging workers through the field or job duties. In addition, the mentor/mentee relationship is one that may last for years, thereby contributing to future socialization for the older person after he or she retires. Furthermore, an older person may develop a legacy through mentoring someone who then becomes successful in a particular field or job. The boot maker is an example of this.

> *Wanjiru Kamau, who immigrated to the United States in 1960 from Kenya, finds her purpose at age 70 in empowering others. She spent several decades back in Kenya working at the University of Nairobi and raising four children. She returned to the United States in 1988 to pursue a doctoral degree, and later worked as an adjunct professor at Penn State University. However, she left academia to become the founder and executive director of African Immigrant and Refugee Foundation. She now helps African immigrants who have struggled to adjust to their new lives. She says, "I find joy in empowering people to solve their problems." Many were refugees; bewildered, illiterate, and unsure of how to find housing or register their children for school. The organization provides African immigrants assistance with mental health services, English classes, tutoring, and cultural clubs for children, and helps resolve conflicts in domestic violence disputes. "My phone rings off the hook at all hours," she says. She works more than 10 hours a day—fielding requests from immigrants, fundraising, and planning for her organization's annual conference. "There are times when money is tight, and I'm up at 3 a.m., that I feel I can't keep up this pace," says Ms. Kamau, who swims and eats a vegetarian diet to stay healthy. "But then I see a child's smile, and I get energized to keep going."*

Dora, age 76, tells this story about her love of work, and how at an early age she learned that earning money empowers:

> *I still go into work and provide a few guest lectures. The extra money from this makes me feel I can spurge on the grandkids. I have also felt empowered, as you say, by working. I will call it independent. As a child I had a strong desire to work. I had numerous start-up "businesses." My earliest memory is selling junk in the kitchen drawer to the neighbors until my mom found out and suggested making and selling potholders. Then I had the idea of organizing talent shows and selling tickets for the shows. This was lots of fun and exposed me to several components of organizing an event. However, I made the most money selling greeting cards. No one could turn me down. I would save my money and then buy something that my parents could not afford to buy me. This gave me some independence at an early age.*
>
> *I could not wait to turn 16, not because I could drive, but because I could work. I learned a lot about myself in that first job, filing credit receipts for a large hardware store. I learned that sitting down all day was not for me and that I did not enjoy being in an environment where I saw the same people every day. Plus, in the break room, people just complained and smoked. What kept me motivated to work was that I had my own money, which gave me freedom of choice, and I could buy things and do activities without asking permission. I paid for my own nursing education, so I could choose where I wanted to go to school.*
>
> *I spent a lot of time with older family members, listening to them talk and observing their lifestyles. It seemed to me that those happiest in their work had some higher education, or at least finished high school, and worked in jobs where they had some autonomy. Each day could be different at their jobs, and there was opportunity to either expand a business or get*

promoted. No one talked about retirement except for those who had health problems or did not like their jobs. I remember one relative, who was still in good health and had a professional job, who was approaching age 65 saying he was not going to retire, as he had nothing else to do: "I will work as long as they will have me."

My own experiences with working or trying as a young child to find work resonated with this idea. I never wanted to be a housewife who stayed at home and worked by myself, wearing a housecoat all day. However, career choices were limited for women. I believed my only options were being a secretary, which required sitting all day so that was not what I wanted, or teaching, which was in a closed environment where the students changed each year, but not the employees. Or I could become a nurse. This seemed at the time to be a good fit because the patients and their families were new, different, and challenging, and nurses seemed to move around from floor to floor. I still would be wearing a housecoat of sorts! So I went to nursing school. I worked in a dynamic teaching hospital. The field of nursing was changing and I changed with it, getting a master's degree in nursing. I started teaching at a community college, providing guest lectures. After a while, I decided that aging nurses do not do well because lifting patients becomes more and more difficult, and I wanted more flexibility in my work schedule because I had three children, so I made the switch to full-time nurse educator. I taught student nurses for over 30 years at the community college, and then at a state university. I retired because the job started to change to doctorate education for faculty and I did not want to go back to school because I had grandkids who needed me. There are actually many professors in nursing education that are over age 65. There is a shortage of us and we feel needed. I am invited back each year to give a couple of guest lectures. I talk about the history of nursing care, as I have not really kept up with all the new technology in medicine. I also provide a lecture on professional nursing behavior. Some of this information does not change! I still keep my nursing R [registration] and belong to my national and state organizations. I love being engaged in nursing education and the students like my stories. I feel young being around them. They ask good questions and this keeps me on my toes. As my relative said, "I hope I can continue to do this for as long as they will have me."

SOCIALIZATION

Quality social contacts are generally beneficial for well-being. Being in a work environment provides social contacts with coworkers and a sense of belonging. Today, grown children and other family members may not live near their older relatives. Consequently, relationships at work become more important, and retirement may lead to social exclusion. As older workers retire, they lose connections because they are no longer in the mix of daily "goings on" in the work environment. Coworkers, who had the work environment as a common bond, may not relate to a retired coworker. The retired person may not want to hear about all the work-related issues anymore, and those still employed may not want to hear about the retired person's daily activities. The retired person may feel excluded when the common bond of work is no longer there. Finally, those working into old age may experience declining health. It may be the social support that they receive at work that becomes critical for their well-being and continued longevity. It may be a coworker who provides a ride to work when the older person's car is being repaired, who brings groceries to the house when the person is ill, or who invites the older person to a family dinner during the holidays.

For older workers, the jobs that are in demand are highly social, and include education, financial services, health care, and consultants, where expertise developed over the life span and professional experience are required (Coombes, 2012). When an older person starts a new job, it opens opportunities to create new relationships. Often, the older worker will become part of this new work community, and make friends with younger workers. This opens up opportunities to engage in fresh perspectives.

MOTIVATIONS FOR WORKING IN RETIREMENT

AARP conducted a nationwide telephone survey of 2,001 individuals between the ages of 50 and 70 years old who are employed on a full-time or part-time basis, in order to better understand the specific types of jobs that workers envision holding in retirement, explore today's definition of retirement, and learn more about the workplace experiences and desires of current working retirees. The phone interviews, which were conducted by Roper ASW using random digit dialing, took place from April 9 through June 5, 2003. Of the individuals interviewed, more than 8 in 10 (85%) had never retired from a job; 15% reported that they had retired from a job, but either remained in the workforce after retiring or had since returned to the workforce.

Although the age of 65 has customarily been associated with retirement, suggesting that the large Baby Boomer cohort (those born between 1946 and 1964) began to leave the workforce in 2011, this AARP study and previous research indicate otherwise. For example, in a 2002 AARP survey of 50- to 70-year-old investors, about 1 in 5 (21%) of investors who had not yet retired reported that they had already postponed retirement as a result of stock market losses, and many of them indicated that they would not retire before the age of 70. Moreover, in this latest study, nearly 70% of workers who had not yet retired reported that they planned to work into their retirement years or never retire, and almost half indicated that they envisioned working into their 70s or beyond.

When asked why they have decided to work in their retirement years, pre-retirees and working retirees were *initially* more likely to identify nonfinancial reasons than financial considerations. Staying "mentally and physically" active and remaining "productive or useful" topped the list. However, when respondents were forced to select only one major factor in their decision to work, it became clear that the "need for money" is the primary motivator. Specifically, when asked to choose only one major influence in their decision to work, both pre-retirees and working retirees were more likely to cite the need for money than any other factor (AARP, 2003).

Interestingly, both pre-retirees and working retirees placed great emphasis on keeping mentally active, with more than 7 in 10 rating this as "very important" in retirement work. In fact, more than half of respondents rated each of the following attributes as "very important" in a retirement job (AARP, 2003):

- Keeps you mentally active; makes you feel useful

- Is fun or enjoyable

- Keeps you physically active

- Enables you to support yourself and your family

- Lets you interact with other people

- Lets you help other people

- Is not too stressful

Allison is a student in a graduate gerontology program, where a course discussion grew about employment and older adults. Allison said that when her mother retired at age 60, she became mentally less sharp. Her memory seemed impaired. Allison would tell her mother a story, and later her mother would tell Allison that someone else told her the story as she repeated it back to Allison. Furthermore, when Allison told her mother that she was going away for the weekend, upon her return, her mother did not remember that Allison had been away. Allison suggested that her mother go back to work part-time because she was also noticing boredom and possible depression in her mother from lack of purposeful activity. Allison relates this story:

> *My mother followed the typical path in life. She graduated from high school and went to college, got married, and then got a job in her field of language and speech pathology. Those working in the school system frequently talked about retirement, and most of my mother's coworkers retired at the same time she did, at age 60. This was the first year that retirement benefits were accessible. My mother never developed hobbies and interests. During the summer months, when my mother did not work in the school system, she would spend time at the pool or shopping. When she retired 2 years ago, there was no structure to her time or how the day was being spent. She filled her time with shopping and meeting with other retired coworkers.*

Allison is also studying occupational therapy, and recognized that her mom needed to have an obligation each day. Her mom's life had become purposeless. She became agitated, high-strung, and nervous.

The school district approached her mom with a part-time job offer. However, she believed working was bad for her health, saying "that is what [she] heard." The other reason was that she "needed to make way for the new employees."

"It was a Public Employees Retirement System mentality," Allison reported. Allison pointed out to her mom that she was not as mentally sharp as when she was working, and that maybe working part-time would be best for her. It took her mom a while to make the decision to go back to work. She had to think about it and realize for herself that she needed to have routine and purpose in her life.

> *When she returned to work, she actually took on new job responsibilities and had to learn new information and processes the first week. It seemed stressful at first, but by the second week she was more comfortable with everything. It was not about money. Having to relearn new job skills seemed to really perk up her cognition. At first the learning was stressful, but then she loved it.*

Conclusion

The Health and Retirement Study, a nationally representative survey of older Americans funded by the National Institute on Aging, has been asking respondents how likely they are to work past ages 62 and 65. Among workers ages 51 to 56, the average expected probability of working full-time past age 62 reached 51% in 2004, up from 47% in 1992. The average expected probability of working full-time past age 65 increased faster, growing from 27 to 33% between 1992 and 2004. Statistical analysis indicated that the declining availability of retiree health benefits, increasing levels of educational attainment, and decreasing traditional pension coverage accounted for most of the increase in work expectations (Mermin, Johnson, & Murphy, 2006). This chapter argues that continued employment adds additional benefits, including providing purpose, empowerment, and socialization, which are all important for wellness and continued quality of life. Currently, there are many publications that advocate diet, exercise, socialization, and cognitive stimulation to age successfully. Being employed in an occupation that one loves encompasses all these wellness recommendations. In addition, working provides purpose and better financial security, which also adds to health. Examples include 87-year-old Azriel Blackman, who has no plans to retire. He was 16 when he started as an apprentice mechanic in 1942 for American Airlines; 70 years later, he still reports to work every day at American's aircraft maintenance hangar at John F. Kennedy International Airport.

> *I don't consider it work, really; if you like what you do, it's not work. My dear wife, when she was alive, used to tell me, "Go to work, bum, go play with your friends."* (Matthews, 2012)

Helen Gurley Brown started *Cosmopolitan* magazine and worked as editor of the American edition until age 75 (Wilson, 2012). She grew up poor and took care of ill family members while growing up. She was an exception for her generation because she earned a business degree and sought out opportunities for success. She died at age 90, and once suggested to *Newsday* that her tombstone should read simply, "She worked very hard." This is the generation that worked through the Depression and World War II. They knew what it meant not to work, the value of working, and did not want to relinquish it. It will be interesting to see what the Baby Boomers' legacy will be because many had the initial goal of early retirement. Now that time is here, and the reality is setting in regarding what life without some type of employment would be like.

REFERENCES

Alexander, C., Langer, E., Newman, R., Chandler, H., & Davies, J. (1989). Transcendental meditation, mindfulness, and longevity: An experimental study with the elderly. *Journal of Personality and Social Psychology, 57*(6), 950-964.

American Association of Retired Persons. (2003). *The AARP Working in retirement study.* Washington, DC: AARP.

Ashenfelter, O., & Card, D. (2001). Did the elimination of mandatory retirement affect faculty retirement flows? National Bureau of Economic Research. Retrieved January 13, 2013, from http://www.nber.org/papers/w8378.

Bourke-White, M. (1963). *Portrait of myself.* New York: Simon and Schuster.

Butler, R. N. (1975). Why survive? Being old in America. New York: Harper & Row.

Calvo, E., Sarkisian, N., & Tamborini, C. R. (2013). Causal effects of retirement timing on subjective physical and emotional health. *Journals of Gerontology Series B: Psychological Sciences and Social Sciences, 68*(1), 73-84.

Committee for Economic Development, Research and Policy Committee. (1999). New opportunities for older workers. New York: Author. Retrieved December 21, 2012, from http://www.ced.org/docs/report/report_older.pdf.

Coombes, A. (2012). For older workers, here is where the jobs will be. *The Wall Street Journal.* Retrieved January 25, 2013, from http://online.wsj.com/article/SB10000872396390443854204578060534215611750.html.

Denmark, F. L., & Williams, D. A. (2012). The older woman as sage: The satisfaction of mentoring. *Women & Therapy, 35*(3-4), 261-278. Retrieved January 1, 2013, from http://dx.doi.org/10.1080/02703149.2012.684543.

Gruenewald, T. L., Liao, D. H., & Seeman, T. E. (2012). Contributing to others, contributing to oneself: Perceptions of generativity and health in later life. *The Journals of Gerontology, Series B: Psychological Sciences and Social Sciences, 67*(6), 660-665.

Hormats, R. (2012). The aging population: Economic growth and global competitiveness. *The Reporter, 4*(4), 10-11.

James, J. B., Besen, E., Matz-Costa, C., & Pitt-Catsouphes, M. (2010). Engaged as we age: The end of retirement as we know it? The Sloan Center on Aging & Work at Boston College. Issue Brief 24. Retrieved January 17, 2013, from https://www.bc.edu/content/dam/files/research_sites/agingandwork/pdf/publications/IB24_EngagedAsWeAge.pdf.

Johnson, R. K. C. (2010). The value of the longtime professor. *New York Times.* Retrieved January 13, 2013, from http://www.nytimes.com/roomfordebate/2010/08/15/aging-professors-who-wont-retire/the-recession-and-the-aging-professor.

June, A. W. (2012). Aging professors create a faculty bottleneck. *The Chronicle of Higher Education.* Retrieved February 24, 2014, from http://chronicle.com/article/Professors-Are-Graying-and/131226/.

Matthews, K. (2012). Airline mechanic with 70-year career has no plans to retire. Retrieved January 26, 2013, from http://www.komonews.com/news/offbeat/Airline-mechanic-Azriel-Blackman-with-70-year-career-has-no-plans-to-retire-163048126.html.

Mermin, G. B. T., Johnson, R. W., & Murphy, D. (2006). *Why do Boomers plan to work so long?* Washington, DC: The Urban Institute. Retirement Project Discussion Paper. Retrieved from http://www.urban.org/url.cfm?ID=311386.

Michels, S. (2013). California Governor Jerry Brown Interview on PBS NewsHour: Balancing the State Budget–1/15/13. Retrieved January 21, 2013, from http://uneditedpolitics.com/california-governor-jerry-brown-interview-on-pbs-newshour-balancing-the-state-budget-11513/.

Moen, P., Erickson, W., Agarwal, M., Fields, V., & Todd, L. (2000). The Cornell Retirement and Well-Being Study. Ithaca, NY: Bronfenbrenner Life Course Center at Cornell University. Retrieved February 24, 2014, from http://worlddatabaseofhappiness.eur.nl/hap_bib/freetexts/moen_p_2000.pdf.

Pitt-Catsouphes, M., & Smyer, M. A. (2006). How old are today's older workers? Retrieved January, 16, 2013, from http://www.agingsociety.org/agingsociety/links/howold.pdf.

Rowe, J.W., & Kahn, R.L. (1997). Successful aging. *The Gerontologist. 37*(4), 433-440.

Silverman, R. E. (2012). The Yankee king of cowboy boots. *Wall Street Journal.* Retrieved January 14, 2013, from http://online.wsj.com/article/SB10001424052970204257504577151404277248024.html.

Stine-Morrow, E. A. L., Parisi, J. M., Morrow, D. G., & Park, D. C. (2008). The effects of an engaged lifestyle on cognitive vitality: A field experiment. *Psychology and Aging, 23*(4), 778-786.

Sullivan, R. (2012). Test of time. *Vogue.* August 2012.

University of Michigan. (2012). Health and Retirement Study, 1992–2008. Retrieved February 28, 2013, from http://hrsonline.isr.umich.edu/.

Wåhlin, I., Ek, A., & Idvall, E. (2010). Staff empowerment in intensive care: Nurses' and physicians' lived experiences. *Intensive & Critical Care Nursing, 26*(5), 262-269.

Wilson, C. (2012). Helen Gurley Brown made 'Cosmopolitan' more than a magazine. Retrieved January 26, 2013, from http://usatoday30.usatoday.com/life/people/obit/story/2011-08-02/helen-gurley-brown-cosmopolitan-dies-at-90/57039456/1.

7

Ergonomics and the Older Person

Jeff Snodgrass, PhD, MPH, OTR/L

Old minds are like old horses; you must exercise them if you wish to keep them in working order.—John Adams (n.d.)

The older worker faces myriad challenges in order to remain a productive member of the workforce. As a person ages, he or she faces increased risk for injury and illness, involuntary job loss, and job opportunities that diminish exponentially with age. In addition, the older worker is faced with increased risk of career-ending disability, increased health insurance costs, as well as concerns regarding health and income security systems, including Social Security, Medicare, retirement accounts, and pensions (Reno & Eichner, 2000). This chapter provides an overview of several topics, including the national work-related injury statistics among older workers in the United States, basic principles of ergonomics and its applications, connection of age-related system changes (physical, vision, hearing, cognitive, and psychosocial) with risk factor assessment of older workers, and ergonomic controls or interventions for reducing hazards in the workplace. It concludes with an interview of an older worker that highlights and brings a personal voice to the chapter's content.

The older person experiences systems changes with age, including physiological, cardiovascular, musculoskeletal, vision, hearing, and cognition (see Chapters 2 and 4). This, in turn, presents challenges in the workplace for older workers, employers, and society in order to keep older workers healthy and productive. However, older workers do not seem to be deterred by these challenges. The Bureau of Labor Statistics (BLS) (2012) estimates that by 2020, when the Baby Boomers move entirely into the 55-years-and-older age group, they will increase their share of the labor force from 19.5% in 2010 to 25.2% in 2020. Interestingly, the working group (ages 25 to 54) typically seen as the "prime age" is projected to drop to almost 64% of the 2020 labor force. Therefore, the older worker is, and will continue to be, a critically important part of the U.S. workforce for years to come.

Hunt LA, Wolverson C.
Work and the Older Person: Increasing Longevity and Well-Being (pp 75-88).
© 2015 SLACK Incorporated.

The reality for many older Americans is their need to continue working well beyond the typical retirement age of 65. In 2007, older men living alone had a median income of $22,300, compared to $34,000 for men under 65. Older women had a median income of $16,000, which was roughly half of that for women under 65 at $30,000. Furthermore, unless a significant change is made to the current Social Security system, it is estimated that retirees (65 years old and older) should expect to receive decreasing net wage replacement from Social Security in the coming decades, compared to retirees over the last 25 years (Reno & Veghte, 2010). Compared to other industrialized countries, older Americans have higher rates of poverty and lower levels of wage-replacement from Social Security. A survey conducted by the American Association of Retired Persons (AARP) found that 78% of workers over 50 years of age that are working or looking for work are doing so primarily due to financial reasons, with only 19% working or looking for work due primarily to nonfinancial reasons, such as "enjoyment or the desire to be productive" (AARP, 2012, p. 1). Therefore, older workers will continue to have strong financial motivation to work beyond the age of 65. Moreover, as noted in several other chapters in this book, the older worker is motivated by a number of additional factors (e.g., self-worth, social engagement) to remain a productive member of the labor force.

This chapter will focus on ergonomic-related issues for the older worker as a strategy to increase the older worker's productivity and longevity in the workforce. The chapter will begin with an overview of national trends in work-related injuries and workers' compensation, describe basic ergonomic principles, proceed to explore age-related system changes with respect to the identification of ergonomics-related risk factors and risk factor assessment, and provide recommendations to accommodate these age-related changes. Ergonomic considerations, from risk factors to interventions/application, will be presented, including physical, cognitive, and environmental factors, job training, and organizational environment.

WORK-RELATED INJURIES, WORKERS' COMPENSATION, AND THE OLDER WORKER

The National Academy of Social Insurance estimates the annual workers' compensation benefits paid for all compensable injuries and illnesses in 2010 at $58 billion (2012). The Liberty Mutual Research Institute reports the direct cost of the most disabling workplace injuries in 2009 to be $50 billion (2011).

Older workers are at a higher risk for compensable work-related injuries and illnesses compared to the entire population. In fact, according to the BLS (2011), older workers (age 65 and over) working in private industry required the longest amount of time to recover from an injury or illness, with a median of 15 days away from work, compared to the average of 8 days away from work for all ages. For older workers in state government and local government jobs, the median days away from work were 19 and 22, respectively, compared to all ages at 10 and 8, respectively. Paradoxically, the incidence rate for musculoskeletal disorders among older workers was 18.3 per 10,000 workers, compared to 34.3 per 10,000 workers for all ages. The top three events or exposures leading to injury or illness in the workplace for older adults were (in descending order) fall on same level, contact with objects or equipment, and overexertion, which includes lifting, pushing, pulling and carrying (BLS, 2011).

Aging predisposes the older worker to an increased risk of workplace injury or illness due to impairments such as hearing loss, decreased vision, cardiovascular compromise, and arthritis, to name a few. The aging workforce will continue to place increased demands on the state-based workers' compensation system. Older people receive a disproportionate amount of Social Security disability benefits, in part due to work-related injuries and illnesses, compared to younger workers (Reno & Eichner, 2000). Given the burgeoning population of older Americans, the number of projected older workers in the years to come, and the high rate of injury among older workers, it is clear that an injury and illness prevention program that includes ergonomics is essential. Applying ergonomic principles to the workplace can lead to the proper identification and abatement of hazards, leading to a safer and friendlier workplace environment for the older worker (Occupational Safety and Health Administration [OSHA], 2012). The next section will provide an overview of basic ergonomics as it relates to identifying and reducing hazards (risk factors) among older workers, followed by a section on age-related systems changes germane to the work setting.

ERGONOMICS

The Basics

Ergonomics is the scientific discipline that deals with the worker; the tools, equipment, and machines that the worker uses; and the environment in which the worker interacts and operates (Annis & McConville, 2012). The literature includes numerous definitions of ergonomics. A holistic definition that best captures the broad scope of ergonomics is provided by the International Ergonomics Association:

> Ergonomics (or human factors) is the scientific discipline concerned with the understanding of the interactions among humans and other elements of a system, and the profession that applies theoretical principles, data and methods to design in order to optimize human well-being and overall system performance. (International Ergonomics Association, 2012, para. 1)

The objective of the application of ergonomics is to fit the work to the worker rather than fit the worker to the work. The outcome of applying ergonomics to the workplace is similar to the outcome of a wellness and health promotion program. The notion of fitting the work to the worker is to minimize, if not eliminate, hazards in the workplace. An analogy can be drawn to reducing an individual's cholesterol through diet and exercise in order to reduce, if not eliminate the hazard of cardiovascular disease. By utilizing a holistic approach using physical, cognitive, and organizational ergonomics, employers create a culture of wellness and health that can lead to improved productivity and increased job satisfaction among older workers, while reducing operational costs and workers' compensation claims (OSHA, 2012; Popkin, Morrow, Di Domenico, & Howarth, 2008; Schwerha & McMullin, 2002). OSHA (2012) estimates that employers who implement an injury and illness prevention program will reduce injuries by up to 35%.

The basic elements of an ergonomic injury prevention program include management leadership (employer), worker participation, hazard identification and assessment, hazard prevention and control, education and training, and program evaluation and improvement (Bush, 2012; OSHA, 2012). All of these program components are essential for an effective and comprehensive injury prevention program. For purposes of this chapter, the focus will be on hazard identification and assessment, prevention and control, and education and training for the older worker.

Hazard Identification and Assessment

Hazard identification and assessment requires the evaluator to perform 2 overarching tasks (Grant, 2012):

1. Review of employer's history of injuries and accidents, employee turnover, as well as review of injury records, e.g., OSHA log of work-related injury and illness (OSHA 300 log), accident reports, and workers' compensation claims, dispensary logs.

2. Assessment of job tasks, processes, tools, and equipment in each work area.

Within these, assessment tasks are discrete activities that must be performed in order to identify the potential hazards (Grant, 2012). General assessment strategies include records review, facility "walk-through" with direct observations, measurements using various tools (e.g., tape measure, force gauges and spring scales, stopwatches), interviews with employers and employees, administration of symptom surveys, various checklists to quantify the extent of exposure to hazards, and generally spending time directly observing the various work areas and workers performing their assigned duties.

An ergonomic hazard identification and assessment considers the following dimensions when identifying potential risk factors:

- *Forceful exertions:* Forces required for lifting, pushing, pulling, carrying, or throwing objects. For example, the requirement to frequently lift and carry boxes weighing 50+ pounds, such as required in the receiving department of a distribution warehouse.

- *Awkward postures:* Awkward postures include positions of the body that are well beyond the neutral range of joints. For example, excessive bending of the back when picking up objects, overhead reaching while painting, wrist flexion while typing on a laptop, squatting and crawling for carpentry work, and neck rotation and flexion while viewing a computer monitor.

- *Repetitive motions:* Motions of the joints that are required frequently throughout the day, such as frequent gripping and pinching required by small parts assembly and excessive wrist flexion and extension with use of a computer mouse.

- *Temperature:* Exposure to cold or hot air and temperatures, and contact with tools that have thermal conductivity (e.g., metal hand tools). For example, a worker in a factory setting where the temperatures exceed 90° Fahrenheit during the summer, or a utility lineman who must work outside in extreme temperatures during the winter months.

- *Vibration:* Exposure to whole body or segmental vibration. The worker may be exposed to vibration through his or her hands, feet, or buttocks. For example, an over the road truck driver is exposed to full body vibration. An example of segmental vibration is a mechanic who uses power hand tools (Griffin, 2012).

- *Other nuisance/environmental factors (noise, micro-shock illumination, color):* A variety of environmental and nuisance factors can contribute to workplace injury and illness. Noise exposure in the workplace has long been recognized as a primary cause of hearing loss (Grinshpun, Kim, & Murphy, 2012). Lighting is important in any work environment, and inadequate or improper lighting can lead to a variety of unsafe working conditions (Bush, 2012). Exposure to chemicals, radiation, and other biologic materials can have deleterious effects on the health of workers.

- *Contact/mechanical stress:* A number of direct contact stress issues may arise in the workplace related to excessive force, weight of a limb on surface, force to operate a tool, and direct contact of a body part on a work surface. Examples of contact stress include direct pressure on the anterior wrists and forearms as an assembly worker rests his hand and forearm on the edge of a table top, or a long-haul truck driver resting his elbow on the center console for prolonged periods.

- *Organizational and psychosocial factors*: A variety of organizational and psychosocial factors can contribute to an unsafe and unhealthy work environment, especially over time. Included in this category are long work hours, shift work, temporal design of work tasks, monotonous work, incentive pay, ability to make decisions and influence working conditions, and interpersonal dynamics, including interactions with coworkers and supervisors (Melin, 2012).

Hazard Prevention and Control

Once ergonomic hazards have been assessed and identified, hazard control and prevention efforts must be undertaken in order to eliminate or reduce identified hazards, including changes and modifications to the process, work methods and tasks, workstations, equipment, and work organization policies (Bush, 2012; OSHA, 2012). Hazard control and prevention efforts are generally focused on one or more of the following categories:

- *Work practice controls:* Examples include modifications of work methods, such as proper body mechanics (e.g., lifting techniques, pacing, employee conditioning, including stretching before and during shift) and job coaching. This category includes education and training of workers with approaches such as continuing education courses to enhance job performance, safety seminars, and on-the-job training.

- *Engineering controls:* This category is considered the most effective hazard control, and includes workstation redesign; modification of tools and equipment to better fit the worker; purchase of new equipment; use of hydraulic lifts, rolling carts, and suspended heavy hand tools; and increasing size of tool handles.

- *Administrative controls:* This includes organizational policies and procedures related to shift work, overtime, rest breaks, number of employees assigned to a task or job, mandatory retirement age, authority and responsibility, productivity rates, equipment maintenance, incentive pay, light duty, restricted duty, and job rotation.

- *Personal protective equipment:* Although not technically an ergonomic control measure, this category includes various protective equipment, such as gloves, respirators, chemical aprons, hard hats, eye protection, ear plugs, steel-toed footwear, and protection against cold, vibration, and contact stress.

The next section will address ergonomics hazard identification and assessment based on typical age-related system changes among older workers.

Age-Related System Changes

This section examines age-related system changes that need to be considered as part of an ergonomic risk assessment. As noted in the previous section, a number of issues, factors, and considerations must be included in identifying risk factors for all workers. In addition, the older worker presents with unique challenges due to age-related system changes, including declines across multiple systems such as cognitive, physical, cardiovascular, visual, hearing, psychomotor, and psychosocial (see Chapter 4). This is further complicated by the reality that older workers may experience a higher incidence of accumulated chronic disorders and conditions, including cardiovascular disease, eye disorders, general orthopedic conditions, diabetes, osteoarthritis, skin disorders, and hearing loss (Association of Occupational and Environmental Clinics, 2009; Gillin, Salmoni, & Shaw, 2008; Hansson, Killian, & Lynch, 2004). Consequently, older workers are often at risk of injuries due to both internal causes (e.g., age-related system changes and general illnesses) and the environmental factors noted in the previous section. This section will attempt to provide the reader with a basic understanding of the age-related system changes that place older workers at a higher risk for work-related injuries and illnesses compared to the entire population (BLS, 2011).

Cognition

The cognitive requirements for work can vary greatly depending on the complexity of the work. Measuring cognitive function and assessing age-related cognitive changes are difficult at best (Skirbekk, Loichinger, & Weber, 2012). Cognitive functioning includes working memory, attention to task, reasoning, and spatial abilities (Pak & McLaughlin, 2011). Cognitive demands are often overlooked when identifying workplace hazards for the aforementioned reasons, but they are especially important to measure with older workers because the literature has consistently identi-fied a strong positive predictive relationship between level of cognitive ability and work success (Salthouse, 2012).

The literature on age-related cognitive declines is robust (Kowalski-Trakofler, Steiner, & Schwerha, 2005). Fluid abilities often decline with age, as can be observed with a slowing of information processing. Attention to task, including divided attention, perceiving and process-ing information, and working memory, are all important abilities used to deal with changing and fluid situations (Pak & McLaughlin, 2011; Schwerha & McMullin, 2002). Findings from research indicate that age-related cognitive changes may impact the older worker's ability to complete work tasks safely and effectively (Choi, 2009; Fozard, Vercryssen, Reynolds, Hancock, & Quilter, 1994; Schwerha & McMullin, 2002). However, it is important to note that research has found that older workers perform well at jobs requiring accumulated or crystallized knowledge because the older worker brings to bear a wealth of experience and expertise in environments with which they are familiar (Kowalski-Trakofler, Steiner, & Schwerha, 2005; Salthouse, 2012). Examples of occupa-tions requiring a high level of fluid abilities include working in a customer service oriented envi-ronment, driving a delivery truck, administrator of an organization, air traffic controllers, and health care workers.

Physical (Including Musculoskeletal)

Most workplace design considerations (i.e., tool design, environmental considerations, job tasks) are based on a "standard" 20- to 40-year-old adult with standard body size and abilities (Kroemer, 2006). The Age Discrimination in Employment Act of 1967 (ADEA) prohibits employ-ment discrimination against persons 40 years of age or older. Although one can argue that older workers often bring experience and perspective to a job, it is also true that as we enter into our 40s and beyond, many physical changes begin to occur.

Research and data highlight a number of physical changes with age (i.e., beyond 40 years of age). The following list includes many of these well documented physical changes, although it is not intended to be exhaustive (Gillin, Salmoni, & Shaw, 2008; Hansson, Killian, & Lynch, 2004; Kjellberg, 2012; Kroemer, 2006):

- Muscle strength deteriorates with a decrease in muscle mass
- Change in articular (joint) surfaces, decreased thickness of joint cartilage, synovial fluid decreases
- Bone density declines (bone brittleness)
- Increase in reaction time and decreased ability to control submaximal forces
- Reduced skin elasticity
- Balance and postural stability decreases that create instability
- Diminished mobility, including walking, standing for prolonged periods, crouching and squatting, kneeling, and climbing
- Decreased elasticity of soft tissue, including stiffness of muscles, tendons, and ligaments.
- Chronic conditions such as osteoarthritis

Due to a combination of age-related changes, older workers may experience difficulty perform-ing in jobs characterized by high physical demands, e.g., crouching, squatting, lifting, pushing, pulling, and reaching overhead (Kowalski-Trakofler, Steiner, & Schwerha, 2005). Examples of occupations requiring high levels of physical exertion include laborers; freight, stock, and mate-rial movers; construction workers; factory workers; nursing aides; orderlies; registered nurses; and janitors (BLS, 2011).

Aerobic Capacity

As we age, our maximal aerobic capacity gradually declines. Most research in this area estimates a decline of about 1% per year after 30 years of age. By the time a person reaches the age of 65, his or her maximal aerobic capacity is approximately 70% of someone who is 25 years of age (Tornqvist, 2012). The decreased aerobic capacity with advancing age can significantly diminish an individual's functional capacity and ability to work in jobs that are not sedentary (Huggett, Connelly, & Overend, 2005; Kowalski-Trakofler, Steiner, & Schwerha, 2005). Thus, work that places a high demand on aerobic capacity is more hazardous for older workers.

Understanding the effects of aging on cardiovascular functioning is complicated by the fact that the effects of aging itself are intimately intertwined with the disease process and lifestyle choices that accompany aging (Fleg, 1986). However, a number of cardiovascular changes typically occur, especially for adults who are 65 or older, including a shrinking of the arterial tree, decreasing pulmonary ventilation, and a decline in maximal heart rate. Occupations that place a high demand on the cardiovascular system are similar to occupations that require moderate to heavy physical workloads, such as the occupations mentioned under the "Physical" heading on p. 80.

Vision

Numerous visual system changes as a result of the normal aging process have been well documented. Functional changes in vision typically result in the following (Hansson, Killian, & Lynch, 2004; Kroemer, 2006; Noell-Waggoner, 2004):

- Size reduction of pupils
- Decreased transparency and thickness of lens
- Diminished visual fields
- Reduced color sensitivity
- Decreased ability to adjust focus and adapt to glare or darkness

Hearing

Functional changes in our auditory systems are commonplace as we age. One of the first age-related declines that people experience is a reduction in hearing. Hearing loss is the third most common chronic health problem after hypertension and arthritis for older adults. Normal conversations are between 45 to 60 decibels (dB). Once individuals reach age 60, they can expect their hearing to decline about 1 dB per year (Walling & Dickson, 2012). High-pitched sounds are typically the first to be lost (Pak & McLaughlin, 2011).

Approximately 50% of the potential for age-related hearing loss can be attributed to genetics. However, work-related factors are a major contributing factor to hearing loss. In fact, occupational hearing loss is a critical issue in the occupational health and safety community. According to The National Institute for Occupational Safety and Health (NIOSH), an estimated 30 million workers are at risk for developing irreversible hearing loss due to exposure to high noise levels (Martinez, 2012).

Examples of occupations with exposure to high noise levels include assembly linesman, orchestra conductor, logger, railroad worker, furniture maker, miner, and airport baggage handler (Martinez, 2012).

Psychological and Social

Everyone faces psychosocial challenges as they go through life. Many of these issues persist across the life span, with some of these issues uniquely age-related. Aging adults often struggle with achieving a work and life balance. Specifically, older workers must often balance the demands of their own work with involvement in the lives of their grandchildren, demands of a spouse's work schedule, and care of a spouse or parents (Association of Occupational and Environmental

Clinics, 2009). Other events that create psychosocial challenges in the workplace for the older person include the following (Association of Occupational and Environmental Clinics, 2009; Reno & Eichner, 2000):

- Uncertainty with their ability to continue in the workforce due to declining mobility, stamina, vision, and hearing

- Losing a job at an older age, which can be especially difficult because displaced older workers are less likely to find work than younger workers

- Loss of income and health insurance coverage with the loss of a spouse

- Assuming the role of caregiver for a spouse

- Illness and disease, acute and chronic

- Disability that prevents continued gainful employment

All of these changes can create psychosocial tensions by impacting work productivity, financial security, overall health status, perceived self-worth, social interactions, and the possibility of isolation.

Examples of occupations that impose a high psychosocial demand include assembly lines with high productivity rates, seasonal work with uncertain job security, high-level executive and administrative work such as vice presidents and chief executive officers, and occupations with low control over decision making coupled with high work output (Melin, 2012).

Getting older necessarily creates age-related changes that may directly impact a person's ability to engage in meaningful and productive work (Moyers & Coleman, 2004). It is imperative to understand the synergy between ergonomic hazards in the workplace and age-related changes. The next section will consider an ergonomic approach to the prevention of work-related injuries for the older worker.

ERGONOMIC INTERVENTIONS AND RECOMMENDATIONS FOR AGE-RELATED SYSTEM CHANGES

After identifying age-related systems changes and potential workplace hazards that place older workers at risk for injury, the next step is to develop and implement ergonomic abatement strategies. For instance, the older worker who presents with decreased strength and flexibility may benefit from engineering controls, including a hydraulic lift that eliminates the need to lift heavy weights (forceful exertions) on a routine basis. An older worker with decreased stamina (aerobic capacity and endurance) may benefit from an administrative control of providing micro-rest breaks throughout the day. This section will present ergonomic strategies to reduce, minimize, or eliminate the risk for work-related injuries in the categories of engineering controls, administrative controls, and work practice controls.

Engineering Controls

Engineering controls are widely considered by occupational health and safety professionals to be the most effective category of ergonomic control, albeit more expensive in many instances. This category includes workstation redesign; modification of tools and equipment to better fit the worker; purchase of new equipment; use of hydraulic lifts, rolling carts, and suspension of heavy hand tools; and increasing size of tool handles (U.S. Department of Health and Human Services, National Institute for Occupational Safety and Health, 2007).

The use of computers is ubiquitous at home and at work. Specific recommendations to improve the computer workstation layout and function include: computer magnification, magnifiers,

TABLE 7-1
EXAMPLES OF ENGINEERING CONTROLS FOR COMPUTER WORKSTATIONS

SYSTEM CHANGES	CONTROLS
Physical	<ul><li>Adjustable height counters</li><li>Sit to stand stools</li><li>Sit to stand mobile workstations</li><li>Adjustable keyboard tray</li><li>Alternatively designed keyboard (e.g., larger split keyboard) and mouse (e.g., wheel)</li><li>Foot rest</li><li>Chair with tilt and adjustable backrest with lumbar support</li><li>Auxiliary, full-sized keyboards and monitors if using a laptop as primary computer</li></ul>
Vision	<ul><li>Flat panel display</li><li>Riser or swivel stand for monitor</li><li>Glare screen</li><li>Screen magnifiers</li><li>Screen magnification</li><li>Document holder</li><li>Larger font</li><li>High contrast ratio between light and dark areas of display</li><li>Viewing angle of display directly in front at eye level</li><li>Nonreflecting materials on interior surface to minimize glare</li><li>Supplemental task/desk lighting</li><li>Blinds or drapes to eliminate bright light</li></ul>
Hearing	<ul><li>Evaluation for a hearing aid if appropriate</li><li>Adaptable headset</li><li>Speaker phone</li><li>Text telephone service (TTY) or text relay service (TRS)</li></ul>

adapted headsets and telephones, frequency modulation (FM) field sound systems, color contrast computer screens, sit-to-stand stools in customer service environments, moveable computer workstations (with sitting and standing option), adjustable height counters, and adjustable keyboards (Gillin, Salmoni, & Shaw, 2008, p. 268). Table 7-1 presents recommendations for computer workstation modifications based on age-related system changes.

TABLE 7-2

EXAMPLES OF ENGINEERING CONTROLS FOR LABOR-INTENSIVE WORK RELATED TO LIFTING, PUSHING, PULLING, AND CARRYING

SYSTEM CHANGE	CONTROLS
Physical and aerobic capacity	• Use scissors lift, load lifter, or pneumatic lifter to raise or lower a load • Use wheeled carts • Use turntable on a work surface or cart • Angled shelving • Use of tools such as counterbalanced power tools • Additional handles for better grip • Increase the size of handles for better grip • Hand pallet trucks
Vision and cognition	• Task lighting directly over work being performed • Slippery surfaces well-marked • Handrails to inclined walking areas • Walkways that are free of obstacles • Effective lighting for stairwells • Use of distinct and contrasting textures and shape for controls • Change of size or color (e.g., color-coding schemes) to set off important visual cues or warning signals
Hearing	• Hearing protection • Minimize background distraction noises • Frequency modulation (FM) field sound systems

Numerous equipment and workstation layout modifications can be made to reduce the required amount of forceful exertions, repetitive motions, and awkward postures. Table 7-2 shows engineering controls related to industrial and labor-intensive work.

Administrative (Organizational) Controls

Administrative controls involve examining organizational policies and procedures in order to maximize an employee's productivity while reducing the risk for injury. Targeted policies and procedures include shift work, overtime, rest breaks, number of employees assigned to a task or job, mandatory retirement age, authority and responsibility, productivity rates, equipment maintenance, incentive pay, light duty, restricted duty, and job rotation. For instance, an older worker who may not be able to tolerate working 8-hour shifts due to decreased stamina may benefit from a part-time position that allows her to work several 4- to 6-hour shifts per week. Table 7-3 presents potential changes to policies and procedures to eliminate or minimize injuries to the older worker.

TABLE 7-3
EXAMPLES OF ADMINISTRATIVE CONTROLS THAT ADDRESS ORGANIZATIONAL POLICIES AND PROCEDURES

SYSTEM CHANGES	CONTROLS
Cognition	• Access to training that is adapted appropriate to older workers (e.g., hands-on learning vs. lecture formats, learning that is self-paced, allow increased time to learn, multimedia approach to training) • Educate managers regarding ways to effectively utilize older workers
Physical and aerobic capacity	• Alternate heavy tasks with light tasks. • Provide variety in jobs to eliminate or reduce repetition (i.e., overuse of the same muscle groups). • Reduce periods of stationary work • Transfer from demanding work to less demanding work according to seniority (the older worker serves as mentor to younger colleagues) • Flexible work hours • Provide recovery time (e.g., short rest breaks) • Modify work practices so that workers perform work within their power zone (i.e., above the knees, below the shoulders, and close to the body)
Psychological and social	• Promote continuous improvement of the work processes for all workers and special accommodations for the aging worker • Job matching for best fit • Removal of mandatory retirement ages • Decrease demands of work performance • Increase the older workers' control over tasks • Provide positive performance and promote positive interactions among older workers • Include training geared towards older worker • Offer opportunities for growth and continued career development • Offer mentoring programs (older workers can serve as coaches for on-the-job training of new employees) • Ensure involvement of aging workers in all aspects of the process to gain ownership and input of their unique capabilities and experiences

TABLE 7-4
EXAMPLES OF WORK PRACTICE CONTROLS FOR A VARIETY OF SETTINGS

SYSTEM CHANGE	CONTROLS
Physical and aerobic capacity	• Have older workers learn to work in *midrange* postures and within the *power zone*. *Midrange* postures are those in which the joints of the neck, back, *legs*, arms, and wrists are not bent in extreme positions. The *power zone* is above the knees, below the shoulders, and close to the body. The principle of the *power zone* is that in this area workers have the greatest power to perform heavier work tasks with less bending, stooping, or reaching • Employee conditioning programs geared toward older workers, (e.g., slow stretching).
Vision and hearing	• Periodic vision and hearing screening for the older worker.
Cognition	• Training programs for improving employee conditioning and work technique geared toward the older worker, including hands-on vs. lecture and self-paced formats
Psychological and social	• Job rotation with a variety of work to reduce monotony

Work Practice Controls

Work practice controls address the methods that workers employ to accomplish their work, including use of body mechanics and proper work techniques, as well as the education and training of workers with on-the-job training opportunities, continuing education (e.g., advanced certification), and safety seminars. An example of a work practice control is engaging older workers in ongoing safety training through a combination of didactic (interactive) training sessions, supplemented by self-paced learning to ensure the individual is properly trained and comfortable performing his or her assigned duties.

Table 7-4 provides several examples of work practice controls that are geared toward the older worker.

James (Figure 7-1), age 82, told his story to Dr. Karen Jacobs, professor of occupational therapy at Boston University. He described the small adaptations he has made with advancing age to enable him to continue to function in his worker role.

James was born in 1930 and grew up in Boston. He held many jobs. For example, in high school, he worked as a bus boy on Martha's Vineyard. Later, he was a gas station attendant, a "bobbin boy," and he worked with a weaver in a mill in Connecticut.

In 1951, James enlisted in the U.S. Navy. He went to boot camp and received training in radio school. He was posted on an 85-man tug boat that escorted nine mine sweepers around the Marshall Islands. The tug boat traveled from Korea to Panama, as well as to Alaska and the North Pole.

When James was 25 years old, he went to TV and electronics school under the GI Bill. In 1955, he started working for Phillip's TV in Brookline, MA. In 1969, the store moved to another location in Brookline, and James became the business owner. The store provided repair, sales, and service with a tender loving care approach. James commented, "You get

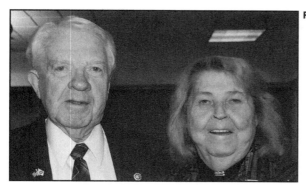

Figure 7-1. James and his wife.

old with them [referring to customers] and they stay loyal to you. Twenty-five years ago, I became an Epson authorized repair store."

James reported that, "I actually do pretty much as I did 40 years ago. I can still carry and move about 50 pounds. Now, I use a dolly and wear glasses. The biggest challenge with being an older worker is hearing, especially with the customers who are non-English speaking. I make eye contact to compensate for my hearing. My memory is starting to go. I know faces and names, but must write them down now. Standing all the time is starting to be problematic. I work 9 to 5 Monday to Friday, and Saturdays from 9 to 1 pm. There are only two people in the store—a technician and me. I am resilient from my childhood. My mom died when I was 12. She was 32 and my dad died at 63. I joined the Brookline Rotary Club in 1984. I am an active member and was a Club president. I am active in the American League Veterans of Foreign Wars, the Shriners, and the Masons. I have been married for over 60 years. I have 4 children and 9 grandchildren. If things were better and if I didn't have stress, I might retire, but I'm not planning to retire because I like people. As long as I stay healthy and keep all of my marbles, I'll keep working."

CONCLUSION

Older workers are a critical part of a productive, sustainable workforce. Workers 55 and older will represent 25% of the labor force by 2020 (BLS, 2012). However, this segment of the workforce presents numerous challenges in order to remain healthy and productive (Reno & Eichner, 2000). It is imperative that robust safety measures and organizational policies are developed and implemented that are tailored to the older worker and include effective ergonomic measures. The application of sound ergonomic principles geared towards the older worker in the workplace can lead to the proper identification and abatement of hazards, leading to a safer and friendlier workplace environment for this burgeoning segment of the labor force (OSHA, 2012).

REFERENCES

Adams, J. (n.d.). Quotes. Retrieved June 12, 2014, from http://www.john-adams-heritage.com/quotes/.

American Association of Retired Persons. (2012). What are older workers seeking? An AARP/SHRM survey of 50+ workers. Retrieved September 3, 2013, from www.aarp.org.

Annis, J. F., & McConville, J. T. (2012). Anthropometry. In A. Bhattacharya & J. D. McGlothlin (Eds.), *Occupational ergonomics: Theory and applications* (2nd ed.). Boca Raton, FL: CRC Press.

Association of Occupational and Environmental Clinics. (2009). Health aging for a sustainable workforce: A conference report. Retrieved September 3, 2013, from http://www.elcosh.org/document/1684/d000987/Healthy%2BAging%2Bfor%2Ba%2BSustainable%2BWorkforce.html.

Bureau of Labor Statistics. (2011). Nonfatal occupational injuries and illnesses requiring days away from work, 2010. Retrieved September 3, 2013, from http://www.bls.gov/iif/oshcdnew.htm.

Bureau of Labor Statistics. (2012). Employment projections 2010-2020. Retrieved September 3, 2013, from http://www.bls.gov/emp.

Bush, P. M. (2012). *Ergonomics: Foundational principles, applications, and technologies.* Boca Raton, FL: CRC Press.

Choi, S. D. (2009). Safety and ergonomic considerations for an aging workforce in the US construction industry. *Work, 33*(3), 307-315.

Fleg, J. (1986). Alterations in cardiovascular structure and function with advancing age. *The American Journal of Cardiology, 57*(5), 33C-44C.

Fozard, J. L., Vercryssen, M., Reynolds S. L., Hancock, P. A., & Quilter, R. E. (1994). Age differences and changes in reaction time: Baltimore longitudinal study of aging. *Journal of Gerontology: Psychological Sciences, 49*, 179-189.

Gillin, E. K., Salmoni, A., & Shaw, L. (2008). Ergonomics of aging. In K. Jacobs (Ed.) *Ergonomics for therapists* (3rd ed.) (pp. 265-276). St. Louis, MO: Mosby Elsevier.

Grant, K. A. (2012). Job analysis. In A. Bhattacharya & J. D. McGlothlin (Eds.), *Occupational ergonomics: Theory and applications* (2nd ed.) (pp. 273-292). Boca Raton, FL: CRC Press.

Griffin, M. J. (2012). Occupational human vibration. In A. Bhattacharya & J. D. McGlothlin (Eds.), *Occupational ergonomics: Theory and applications* (2nd ed.) (pp. 765-790). Boca Raton, FL: CRC Press.

Grinshpun, S. A., Kim, J., & Murphy, W. J. (2012). Noise exposure and control. In A. Bhattacharya & J. D. McGlothlin (Eds.), *Occupational ergonomics: Theory and applications* (2nd ed.) (pp. 791-826). Boca Raton, FL: CRC Press.

Hansson, R. O., Killian, J. H., & Lynch, B. C. (2004). The older worker. In M. J. Sanders (Ed.), *Ergonomics and the management of musculoskeletal disorders* (2nd ed.) (pp. 437-447). St. Louis, MO: Butterworth-Heinemann.

Huggett, D. L., Connelly, D. M., & Overend, T. J. (2005). Maximal aerobic capacity testing of older adults: A critical review. *The Journals of Gerontology, 60A*(1), 57-66. Retrieved September 3, 2013, from http://search.proquest.com/docview/208620676?accountid=14872.

International Ergonomics Association. (2014, May 15). Retrieved from http://www.iea.cc/whats/index.html.

Kjellberg, K. (2012). Work requiring considerable muscle force. In A. Toomingas, S. E. Mathiassen, & E. W. Tornqvist (Eds.), *Occupational physiology* (pp. 59-97). Boca Raton, FL: CRC Press.

Kowalski-Trakofler, K. M., Steiner, L. J., & Schwerha, D. J. (2005). Safety considerations for the aging workforce. *Safety Science, 43*, 779-793.

Kroemer, K. H. (2006). Designing for older people. *Ergonomics in Design: The Quarterly of Human Factors Applications, 14*(4), 25-31.

Liberty Mutual Research Institute. (2011). 2011 Liberty Mutual workplace safety index.

Martinez, L. F. (2012). Can you hear me now? Occupational hearing loss, 2004-2010. *Monthly Labor Review, 135*(7), 48-55.

Melin, B. (2012). Work with high levels of mental strain. In A. Toomingas, S. E. Mathiassen, & E. W. Tornqvist (Eds.) *Occupational physiology* (pp. 183-213). Boca Raton, FL: CRC Press.

Moyers, P. A., & Coleman, S. D. (2004). Adaptation of the older worker to occupational challenges. *Work, 22*(2), 71-78.

National Academy of Social Insurance. (2012). Workers' compensation: Benefits, coverage, and costs, 2010. Retrieved from http://www.nasi.org/research/2012/report-workers-compensation-benefits-coverage-costs-2010.

Noell-Waggoner, E. (2004). Lighting solutions for contemporary problems of older adults. *Journal of Psychosocial Nursing and Mental Health Services, 42*(7), 14-20.

Occupational Safety and Health Administration (OSHA), 2012. Injury and illness programs. White paper. Retrieved from https://www.osha.gov/dsg/topics/safetyhealth/.

Pak, R., & McLauglin, A. (2011). *Designing displays for older adults.* Boca Raton, FL: CRC Press.

Popkin, S. M., Morrow, S. L., Di Domenico, T. E., & Howarth, H. D. (2008). Age is more than just a number: Implications for an aging workforce in the US transportation sector. *Applied Ergonomics, 39*, 542-549.

Reno, V. P., & Eichner, J. (2000). Ensuring health and income security for an aging workforce. Retrieved September 3, 2013, from http://www.nasi.org.

Reno, V. P., & Veghte, B. (2010). Economic status of the elderly in the United States. Prepared for the National Academy of Social Insurance. Retrieved September 3, 2013, from http://www.nasi.org.

Salthouse, T. (2012). Consequences of age-related cognitive declines. *Annual Review of Psychology, 63*, 201-226.

Schwerha, D. J., & McMullin, D. L. (2002). Prioritizing ergonomic research in aging for the 21st century American workforce. *Experimental Aging Research, 28*, 99-110.

Skirbekk, V., Loichinger, E., & Weber, D. (2012). Variation in cognitive functioning as a refined approach to comparing aging across countries. *Proceedings of the National Academy of Sciences of the United States of America, 109*(3), 770-774.

Tornqvist, E. W. (2012). Work demanding high energy metabolism. In A. Toomingas, S. E. Mathiassen, & E. W. Tornqvist (Eds.), *Occupational physiology* (pp. 19-58). Boca Raton, FL: CRC Press.

U.S. Department of Health and Human Services, National Institute for Occupational Safety and Health (2007). Ergonomic guidelines for manual material handling (Publication No. 2007-131). Retrieved September 3, 2013, from http://www.cdc.gov/niosh/docs/2007-131/.

Walling, A., & Dickson, G. (2012). Hearing loss in older adults. *American Family Physician, 85*(12), 1150-1156.

8

Cognitive Benefits of Working

Ross Andel, PhD

The excitement of learning separates youth from old age. As long as you're learning, you're not old.—Rosalyn S. Yalow (Voorhees, 2001)

Cognitive impairment is arguably the most feared aspect of aging, yet factors influencing the risk of cognitive impairment are still relatively poorly understood. Genetic predisposition, early-life influences, exposure to intellectually stimulating environments, exercise, and dietary factors are all believed to contribute to the variations in risk of cognitive impairment across aging individuals (Andel, Hughes, & Crowe, 2005; Hughes & Ganguli, 2009; Weinstein, Wolf, Beiser, Au, & Seshadri, 2013). Although some portion of cognitive outcomes later in life is attributable to genetic influences and early-life influences beyond the person's control (Gatz, 2005; Salthouse, 2009), there are still important factors that influence the risk in midlife and late life that may be modified. These modifiable factors play a particularly prominent role in research because of their promise to delay the onset of cognitive decline and impairment. However, research has yet to progress to a point where a specific behavior, or behavioral modification, is substantiated enough to be broadly recommended to the public.

Based strictly on length of exposure over the life course, it would be hard to argue against the premise that occupation is a major player amongst the modifying factors that may significantly alter the course of cognitive aging. Only sleep rivals work with respect to the amount of time accumulated in one activity over a lifetime. Research seems to support the notion that occupation plays a crucial role in cognitive functioning and cognitive aging, with most support currently gathered for socioeconomic status, occupational complexity, and work-related stress as important determinants of cognitive aging.

Hunt LA, Wolverson C.
Work and the Older Person: Increasing Longevity and Well-Being (pp 89-100).
© 2015 SLACK Incorporated.

GENETICS AS A FACTOR IN COGNITIVE FUNCTION AND DECLINE

To objectively discuss the cognitive benefits of any potentially modifiable activity including work, genetic predisposition needs to be mentioned. Genetic factors seem to determine around 40% to 80% of cognitive performance (Plomin, 1999), although genetic influence declines somewhat in very old age (Finkel, Reynolds, McArdle, & Pedersen, 2005). Family history and genetic predisposition also play important roles in the risk of developing Alzheimer's disease (Ashford & Mortimer, 2002). In particular, one gene, the APOE e4 allele, has been cited quite consistently as a risk factor for Alzheimer's disease (Poirier, 2000).

Although genetic factors are an important foundation of cognitive resources, there may be modifiable environmental factors that help maintain the existing cognitive reserve and reduce risk of cognitive impairment. Occupation, with its exceptional overall length of exposure and its central role in the lives of most individuals, should be considered one of the central candidates for intervention in this regard. Although occupation may be predetermined by genetic, and potentially also early-life, factors to some extent (Potter, Plassman, Helms, Foster, & Edwards, 2006), there is also evidence indicating that occupational exposure may provide cognitive benefits above and beyond these familial influences (Andel, Crowe, et al., 2005).

Several theories help us understand how these modifiable factors, including occupation, affect cognitive aging. The most prominent among them are the concept of cognitive reserve and the environmental complexity hypothesis. However, the discussion of cognitive aspects of work cannot be carried out properly without considering socioeconomic position, which is inherently tied with one's occupation.

SOCIOECONOMIC POSITION AS A FACTOR IN COGNITIVE FUNCTION AND DECLINE

The effects of cognition are not restricted to individuals themselves, but extend to the work status of the parents. Specifically, parents' socioeconomic position appears to be a good determinant of adulthood cognitive function, with lower parental position being indicative of reliably poorer cognitive performance throughout the life course in the offspring (Kaplan et al., 2001). In addition, having fewer siblings and growing up in the suburbs as opposed to an urban area appear to be associated with lower risk for Alzheimer's disease (Moceri, Kukull, Emanuel, van Belle, & Larson, 2000). These factors seem to reflect socioeconomic influences on brain development that may impact both occupational opportunities and subsequent cognitive outcomes.

Closely tied to childhood socioeconomic status is the amount of education an individual attains. Not surprisingly, education has often emerged as a major predictor of late-life cognitive health (Gatz et al., 2001; Ngandu et al., 2007; Sharp & Gatz, 2011). A recent review suggests that education is particularly pertinent to late-life cognitive outcomes in more developed regions where it is more likely to reflect actual cognitive capacity and less so in less developed regions where it is more likely also tied to opportunity (Sharp & Gatz, 2011).

Finally, adult occupational status has also been linked to cognitive function and status later in life. For example, working in occupations characterized by low socioeconomic status has been found to increase the risk of dementia in studies across the world, including the Canadian Study of Health and Aging (1994), studies based in Sicily (Azzimondi, D'Alessandro, Pandolfo, & Feruglio, 1998), Finland (Anttila et al., 2002), and Sweden (Qui et al., 2003), as well as studies of incident dementia conducted in East Boston (Evans et al., 1997) and New York (Stern et al., 1994).

However, not all studies have confirmed the hypothesis that individuals pay a cognitive price for exposure to low-status occupations. For example, findings from the Illinois-based Religious Orders Study (Wilson et al., 2005) indicate that early life socioeconomic status, although associated with cognitive function, may not capture reliably the differences in rate of cognitive decline or risk of dementia. In addition, no association between low- versus high-status occupation and risk of dementia was reported in case-control studies such as the Conselice Study based in Northern Italy (Ravaglia et al., 2002), the French PAQUID (Personnes Agées QUID) project (Helmer et al., 2001), or a study conducted in the United Kingdom (Paykel et al., 1994).

Finally, there is substantial evidence that differences in work environments influence cognitive aging (Andel, Crowe, Kareholt, Wastesson, & Parker, 2011; Andel, Crowe, et al., 2005; Andel, Kareholt, Parker, Thorslund, & Gatz, 2007; Potter, Helms, Burke, Steffens, & Plassman, 2007). It could also be argued that many work-related factors are more easily modified than someone's education or socioeconomic status.

In the past 2 decades, 2 major hypotheses have emerged as researchers in aging have continued to disentangle the underlying mechanisms of the association between continued engagement in activities that may stimulate the mind and stability of cognitive functioning—the environmental complexity hypothesis (Kohn & Schooler, 1983) and the concept of cognitive reserve (Stern, 2002, 2012).

COGNITIVE BENEFITS OF EXPOSURE TO INTELLECTUALLY STIMULATING WORK ENVIRONMENTS

The Environmental Complexity Hypothesis and the Concept of Cognitive Reserve

Kohn and Schooler (1983) suggested that cognitive functioning in older adults is influenced by the demands of their environments. The central proposition in the environmental complexity hypothesis is that highly complex environments that consistently offer opportunities for participating in self-directed and substantively complex tasks (such as occupations that engage the worker intellectually), increase intellectual flexibility and, subsequently, promote relatively stable cognitive functioning in older adulthood. To substantiate the environmental complexity hypothesis, factor analysis-based scores from self-reports about complexity of work with data, people, and things were derived (Schooler, 1984; Schooler, Mulatu, & Oates, 1999). Results based on this measure provided evidence that substantive complexity of work may facilitate cognitive function among employed adults (Schooler et al., 1999). Empirical work testing this hypothesis later moved to test whether the influence of exposure to complex environments may persist into older adulthood, as would be evidenced by reduced risk of cognitive impairment and dementia.

Several of the work-related factors associated with cognitive function later in life, and particularly socioeconomic status and complexity of work, have been tied to the idea that work offering opportunities for mental exercise and work characterized by low risk of adverse exposure would boost cognition via a positive influence on cognitive reserve. According to the cognitive reserve hypothesis (Stern, 2002, 2012), individual differences in cognitive abilities are linked to underlying differences in the brain neurophysiology and/or the ability to compensate for age-related neuronal damage by superior problem-solving strategies. The characteristics of one's neural substrate, and the ability to use compensatory strategies as the reserve becomes depleted, may determine when or if a person becomes cognitively impaired.

In one particularly interesting study, Stern et al. (1995) measured current cerebral blood flow in relation to work environment in a sample of patients recently diagnosed with Alzheimer's disease. To measure work environment, they used factor scores reflecting substantive complexity, interpersonal demands, management requirements, and physical demands derived from occupational characteristics based on the *Dictionary of Occupational Titles* (U.S. Department of Labor, 1977). They found that patients who had held jobs with high interpersonal and physical demands had relatively greater deficits in cerebral blood flow in the parietal area compared to patients who had held jobs with low demands when dementia severity, age, and education were controlled. Apparently, these patients must have functioned without clinical diagnosis of Alzheimer's disease even while dementia-related neurodegenerative processes were affecting neuronal networks. On the other hand, patients with Alzheimer's disease who had held jobs with lower demands progressed to the diagnosis of Alzheimer's disease at a significantly earlier stage of neurodegeneration. These findings offer direct evidence for the notion that stimulating work environment can support cognitive reserve, delaying the actual clinical onset of dementia.

Several studies have tested the concept of cognitive reserve using measures of occupational complexity derived from the research on environmental complexity (Kohn & Schooler, 1983). One test of the cognitive reserve hypothesis using measures of occupational complexity comes from a longitudinal study conducted with data from the Alzheimer's Disease Research Center at the University of Southern California (Andel, Vigen, Mack, Clark, & Gatz, 2006). The study offers another approach to the examination of the validity of this hypothesis while using patients already diagnosed with Alzheimer's disease, similar to Stern et al. (1995). A total of 139 patients just diagnosed with Alzheimer's disease were followed for about 2.5±2 years to assess the rate of cognitive decline. Occupational complexity was measured as substantive complexity of work and complexity of work with data, people, and things. Average lifetime occupational complexity was calculated based on years at each occupation. The hypothesis was that having had a job with a high level of complexity would lead to a delayed onset of Alzheimer's disease, as evidenced by more widespread brain pathology at the time of diagnosis. The extent of brain pathology was assessed indirectly by change in cognitive scores, expecting greater initial state of pathology to be reflected in a faster rate of cognitive decline. Mixed-effects models were used to properly account for the different number of follow-ups, different intervals between follow-up, and variable starting points with respect to cognitive function.

The stated hypothesis was confirmed with overall (substantive) complexity, as well as complexity of work with data and people. That is, Alzheimer's disease patients who had held jobs with high complexity were showing far steeper decline in their cognitive abilities following diagnosis. The most obvious explanation for this result is that cognitive reserve, facilitated by exposure to complex work environment, acted as a buffer against more rapid decline in important daily functions, including cognitive function, extending dementia-free life to a point at which brain pathology was too substantial. Then, a more precipitous decline followed. This study offers a unique approach to testing the potential cognitive benefits of occupational complexity. A more conventional approach involves exploration of the link between occupational complexity and subsequent cognitive decline or impairment. One such study looked at complexity in main lifetime occupation in relation to risk of dementia in a large, population-based sample of Swedish twins (Andel, Crowe, et al., 2005). One of the advantages was the use of two designs within one study—a classic cohort design and a co-twin control design—that provides an opportunity to test more directly the possibility that the association between occupational complexity and dementia is simply a function of genetic or familial confounding. The main finding of this study was that higher complexity of work with people was linked to lower risk of dementia, and Alzheimer's disease specifically, independent of covariates such as age, sex, and education. The finding that occupational complexity may reduce the risk of dementia was later replicated with data from the Canadian Study of Health and Aging (Kroger et al., 2008) and the Kungsholmen Project (Karp et al., 2009), providing solid evidence for the existence of this association.

Just as importantly, in the study by Andel and colleagues (2005), occupational complexity continued to confer lower risk of dementia when only data for complete twin pairs were used. This is important because it suggests that the association between more complex (stimulating) work environment and lower risk of dementia may exist above and beyond predisposing factors, such as genetic and early-life factors shared by twins. This possibility was supported in a study published 2 years later with data from the National Academy of Sciences-National Research Council Twins Registry of World War II veterans (Potter et al., 2007). Specifically, the authors reported that an association between greater intellectual job demands and lower risk of dementia was observed both among cases and controls that were independent and in between twin pairs where one twin was diagnosed with dementia while the co-twin remained dementia free for at least 6 extra years.

Can Causality Be Determined in the Association Between Work Complexity and Cognitive Outcomes?

One important question in the context of the presented support for the cognitive benefits of high occupational complexity (or another source of intellectual stimulation) is the uncertainty about the direction of this relationship. A possibility has been presented that individuals who are more engaged in intellectually stimulating activities have preselected themselves into this intellectually active group. Thus, any observed effect of such intellectual engagement on cognitive outcomes is a reflection of initially higher levels of cognitive functioning (preserved differentiation), rather than stable cognitive function as a result of continued high levels of intellectual engagement (differential preservation), a common explanation for why occupational complexity or another source of intellectual engagement may relate so consistently to cognitive outcomes (Salthouse, 2006).

A study by Finkel, Andel, Gatz, and Pedersen (2009) offers a somewhat more refined approach to testing the contrast between preserved differentiation and differential preservation with respect to occupational complexity. Finkel and colleagues used a longitudinal assessment of cognitive function, starting at age 50 and continuing through older adulthood, and modeled cognitive change specifically before and after the onset of retirement. Three hypotheses were tested:

1. There would be higher levels of cognitive performance for those with more complex occupations (preserved differentiation)

2. Mental practice offered by complex occupation would lead to differential preservation of cognitive skills, or slower cognitive aging (differential preservation)

3. Retirement would have a more negative impact on cognitive skills in individuals retiring from complex occupations, as previously suggested by Schaie (2005)

Most notably, complexity of work with people indicated differential preservation in verbal memory. That is, individuals engaged in occupations characterized by high complexity of work with people showed continued relative improvements in this domain up until retirement, at which point their cognitive advantage started to dissipate. In addition, following retirement, individuals previously holding jobs with high complexity of work exhibited faster rate of decline, although only on spatial ability. Again, this finding provides evidence for the possibility that exposure to complex environments facilitates cognitive function.

Motivation at Work and Cognitive Health

Recently, the idea has emerged that one's approach to work environment, or motivation, may confer influence on cognitive health and aging. The idea is based on the premise that the will or drive to improve one's skills, and personality traits that underlie it, are reflected in both occupational selection and the approach to work. The effect of occupation would then reflect not only the exposure to a certain work environment (such as occupational demands or complexity), but also inherent characteristics that allow for a certain work environment to have a particular effect on cognitive and other health outcomes. One such study introduces the concept of "motivational reserve" (Forstmeier et al., 2012) as an important predictor of risk of dementia. Specifically, occupational characteristics allowing for self-regulation of skill and the will to better oneself may provide the type of intellectual benefits that are later reflected through a reduced risk of dementia.

The Israeli Ischemic Heart Disease Project offers another interesting take on motivation and cognitive health (Ravona-Springer, Beeri, & Goldbourt, 2013). The authors asked "Do you want to improve your status at work and do you believe it is possible?" of participants during their midlife in relation to risk of dementia assessed 37 years later. The possible answers included (a) trying to change status and believe it is possible, (b) trying but unsure of success, (c) not trying, unlikely to succeed, and (d) not trying, satisfied. The results indicated that, relative to option (a), answering (b), (c), or (d) was related to a significantly increased risk of dementia, with option (d) approximately doubling the risk.

COGNITIVE COSTS OF EXPOSURE TO WORK-RELATED STRESS

It is widely accepted that chronic exposure to stress can have many detrimental health consequences. Several pathways have been suggested for this effect. One frequently cited pathway revolves around the concept of "allostatic load" (McEwen, 1998, 2007). Within this concept, persistent exposure to stress eventually leads to overactivation of the hypothalamic-pituitary-adrenal (HPA) axis and, subsequently, chronic elevation of glucocorticoids (e.g., cortisol), which are designed to provide us with the fight-or-flight response. In other words, exposure to psychological stress "tricks" the body into thinking that a physical threat is present. To correctly respond to this threat, hormones that stimulate systems essential for physical strength and high levels of alertness (i.e., glucocorticoids) are released. Reestablishing optimal physiological balance (i.e., homeostasis or allostasis) takes effort. This effort is captured by allostatic load. This process has been linked to accelerated biological aging (Finch & Seeman, 1999; McEwen, 1998, 2007; Sapolsky, 1996) as well as accelerated brain aging specifically (Kiecolt-Glaser, McGuire, Robles, & Glaser, 2002). The personality trait of neuroticism (Crowe, Andel, Pedersen, Fratiglioni, & Gatz, 2006; Wang et al., 2009) and post-traumatic stress disorder (Yaffe et al., 2010)—both markers of chronic stress—have been associated with cognitive impairment and dementia in later life. Evidence is now emerging indicating that work-related stress may influence risk of dementia in a similar fashion.

In the past 30 or so years, the job strain model (Karasek, 1979; Karasek & Theorell, 1990) has been widely used to capture levels of stress at work. The model states that jobs associated with low job control, high job demands, low social support at work, and the negative combinations of these factors are stressful and lead to poorer health outcomes. Although not all studies find support for this model, there is wide evidence suggesting that differences in work-related stress conveyed by the job strain model are predictive of health problems, particularly cardiovascular disease (Belkic, Landsbergis, Schnall, & Baker, 2004; Eller et al., 2009). Given the proposed connection between risk factors for dementia and risk factors for cardiovascular disease (Launer, 2002), it is no surprise that studies assessing the role of work-related stress in risk of dementia have recently started to emerge.

Initial evidence for the role of work-related stress in risk of dementia comes from a study conducted in Germany using a job exposure matrix, where lack of control over work tasks (as well as lack of intellectual or social demands) conferred greater risk of dementia (Seidler et al., 2004). However, a study using data from the Swedish Twin Registry observed that self-reported high job demands did not reliably differentiate those at risk for dementia, although self-reported reactivity to stress did (Crowe, Andel, Pedersen, & Gatz, 2007).

It is important to point out that the two studies mentioned above did not use theory-based measures of work-related stress. Since then, two studies were published that utilize the theoretical framework proposed by Karasek and Theorell regarding job strain (Karasek & Theorell, 1990). In a study based in Sweden (Wang, Wahlberg, Karp, Winblad, & Fratiglioni, 2012), low control and the combination of low control with high demands (high job strain) were found to increase the risk of dementia. Similarly, a study using data from the Swedish Twin Registry (Andel et al., 2012) reported that lower job control, lower social support at work, and greater job strain (especially when combined with low social support) were all associated with greater risk of dementia. In addition, the association was particularly pronounced for vascular dementia, supporting the notion that work stress may increase the risk of dementia via a cardiovascular pathway.

COGNITIVE EFFECTS OF RETIREMENT

Retirement Transition

Work is considered one of the central tenets of life in modern society. Therefore, retirement needs to be considered a major life transition, with potentially important consequences for cognitive functioning and cognitive aging. The few studies on retirement and cognition point to different, often somewhat conflicting, conclusions, leaving this area of research wide open and in need of additional study. For example, in a large scale, multinational study (Adam, Bonsang, Grotz, & Perelman, 2013), the authors analyzed data from the Survey on Health, Ageing and Retirement in Europe (a dataset that includes more than 25,000 individuals aged 50+ from 11 European countries), and the Health and Aging Study (a population-based ongoing panel survey of health, well-being, retirement, and aging among older adults living in the contiguous United States [Heeringa & Connor, 1995]), to assess the impact of retirement on cognitive functioning. The main conclusion was that retirement, regardless of the job from which individuals retire, at what age they retire, or in which country they live, has adverse consequences for cognitive function. The same conclusion was reached by a similar, earlier study that also included data from England (Rohwedder & Willis, 2010), with the caveat that the negative effect of retirement is particularly visible in the early 60s.

Coe and colleagues (2012) offer a slightly more refined look at retirement and cognition in data collected by the Health and Retirement Survey, and potentially conflicting results. First, using a similar universal approach to data analysis, the authors reported to confirm the negative effect of retirement on cognition, which was modified by retirement duration (longer duration, greater effect). However, they also assessed the possibility of reverse causation, whereby the decision to retire is a consequence of cognitive difficulties. When extraneous variables influencing the decision to retire were taken into account, a strikingly different pattern of results emerged. There was no evidence for the negative association between retirement and cognitive function. In fact, when data were analyzed separately by blue- or white-collar status, there was a positive association between retirement and cognitive function specific to blue-collar workers. The authors speculate that these results are not necessarily contrary to the premise that work activity, or activity in general, would not carry cognitive benefits. Rather, it may be that those retiring from blue-collar jobs may have an easier time finding opportunities for intellectual engagement outside the workplace, whereas the pattern of postretirement activity among white-collar workers may vary too widely for any reliable results to emerge.

Current Trends and Retirement

Recent economic trends (other than higher unemployment), as well as amendments to retirement and health policies, may lead to the postponement of retirement among some workers, particularly those feeling less economically secure (Helman, Greenwald, VanDerhei, & Copeland, 2007; McFall, 2011; Mermin, Johnson, & Murphy, 2007; Szinovacz, Martin, & Davey, 2014). This is a potentially important trend that may need more attention in scientific literature, particularly given that there is currently some disagreement as to whether retirement is a positive or negative event with respect to cognitive functioning. If anything, there are suggestions that retiring later may lead to more favorable late-life outcomes (Calvo, Sarkisian, & Tamborini, 2013). However, the possibility that this effect could be at least partially attributable to better health among those who remain in the workforce (as opposed to those who retire early) cannot yet be discounted.

The social context of work should also be considered. Retirement constitutes a significant life transition that involves planning based on personal preferences, economic resources, and social and policy norms (Ekerdt, Kosoloski, & DeViney, 2000; Szinovacz, Martin, & Davey, in press). Prior to retirement, engagement within one's work context constitutes a key source of identity as well as social relationships, which has far reaching implications for functioning across domains (e.g., Heckhausen, Wrosch, & Schulz, 2010). However, transitioning into retirement signifies disengagement from the workforce and diminishes the possibilities for a wide social network beyond one's family. Due to the significance of retirement, this can have a tremendous impact on one's cognitive and physical health in the years following retirement (Calvo, Sarkisian, & Tamborini, 2013; Ekerdt, 2010; Kim & Moen, 2002).

One compelling argument for the importance of social context at work comes from the study examining the association between work-related stress and risk of dementia using the Swedish Twin Registry (Andel, Crowe, et al., 2005), which was discussed earlier. Specifically, there was a consistent association between work-related stress indicative of low social support from coworkers and supervisors, and greater risk of dementia decades later. In addition, the overall effect of having low control at work in combination with high demands was significantly compounded when the environment also involved low social support. There are at least two ways in which to interpret these findings. First, social support at work provides for a more pleasant work experience, which carries through the retirement years, ultimately reducing the risk of dementia. Alternatively, social relationships established during working years may carry over to retirement. Therefore, the work environment can continue to influence cognitive aging past retirement by providing workers who establish meaningful relationships at work with social resources well past retirement.

Despite these initial findings, the effect of retirement on cognitive function is still not well understood. Given the prolonged period of exposure to the work environment, it is highly likely that work should have an effect on cognitive aging that spans well into postretirement years, as evidenced by prior research with work-related stress and cognitive outcomes (Andel et al., 2011, 2012; Wang et al., 2012), or complexity of work and cognitive outcomes (Andel, Crowe, et al., 2005; Andel et al., 2007; Schooler et al., 1999).

Below, Marie tells her story of the importance of employment to cognitive functioning within her work history.

> *Marie is 72 years of age. She worked for over 30 years as a hospital admitting clerk. "I retired when I was 53 years of age because my husband just reached his legal retirement age. Although my retirement benefits were to be reduced quite significantly, spending time with my now retired husband was a big motivating factor. Plus, this practice was very common among my peers. When the husband retires, the wife retires as well. Unfortunately, my husband died about 6 months after I entered into retirement. This was a shock for a number of reasons, including the fact that all family matters that we used to deal with together now fell squarely on my shoulders. My already slim retirement benefits were reduced even further.*
>
> *Within a year or so, I decided to try to reenter the workforce. While my position was no longer available, I was lucky enough to be hired for a similar position at the same hospital 2 years after my retirement, at age 55. To my great surprise, the 2 years away from this work had a profound influence on my ability to perform at work. Particularly my stamina was a surprisingly great issue. I used to manage my own position while also helping with the tasks of others. Now, I was not even able to effectively complete my own basic tasks. Particularly working in the early afternoon was proving to be very challenging. Retirement offered me the opportunity to take short naps after lunch. My body, now used to these pleasant siestas,*

was refusing to engage in intellectually challenging work activity for at least an hour following lunch time. Instead, I would be falling asleep at my desk. This of course did not bode well with my supervisors or coworkers.

I was never able to readjust to a full-time position after just 2 years of retirement. Therefore, I eventually retired again, this time for good. I really enjoy my retirement now and I would never again attempt to reenter the workforce. I have my routine with lots of time just for myself. I try to stay intellectually active by doing crossword puzzles and other activities that I consider stimulating daily. I also like to watch several TV shows that I believe keep me mentally active.

Looking back, I consider gainful employment extremely important for one's cognitive functioning and for how one ages cognitively. The amount of concentration that is involved can hardly be matched by anything I can do in retirement. Also, since workers are constantly being evaluated, the pressure to perform further stimulates one's cognitive abilities, which is a significant factor in maintaining cognitive skills. This pressure largely disappears after retirement, and so does the need to engage oneself fully in something. I believe this aspect of work environment cannot be replaced.

When do I think may be the right time to retire? This depends on the person's physical and mental health. When health begins to deteriorate, work can be a huge burden. Therefore, early retirement would be the perfect solution. However, for a healthy person, the best time to retire would certainly be some time in their 60s. Even late 60s would probably work well. I retired much too early.

CONCLUSION

Work is one of the central tenets of human life. In general, time spent at work is rivaled only by time spent sleeping. Therefore, the fact that more and more research points to the influence of work environment on health and aging (including cognitive aging) is not surprising. Genetic and early-life environmental factors affect job selection, establishing certain patterns for late-life cognitive outcomes. Still, there are several aspects of the work environment that relate to cognitive health in older adulthood, above and beyond genetics and childhood environment. These include complexity of work and work-related stress. Specifically, complexity of work, particularly complexity of work with data and people, provides measurable benefits for cognitive health, whereas work-related stress, particularly lack of job control, lack of social support, and the combination of low job control/high job demands, adversely affect cognitive health. Therefore, efforts should be made to find meaningful roles and opportunities for engaging the worker, particularly for positions where such opportunities are not obvious. Finally, given the importance of work in human society, retirement represents a major life transition that should be taken into account as a potentially critical factor with respect to cognitive aging. There is some evidence suggesting that retirement can adversely affect cognitive aging, although evidence for this statement is still questionable, particularly for those retiring from blue collar jobs. Improving our understanding of work environment and retirement can help expand cognitive benefits of working and is therefore a worthwhile effort.

REFERENCES

Adam, S., Bonsang, E., Grotz, C., & Perelman, S. (2013). Occupational activity and cognitive reserve: Implications in terms of prevention of cognitive aging and Alzheimer's disease. *Clinical Interventions in Aging, 8,* 377-390.

Andel, R., Crowe, M., Hahn, E. A., Mortimer, J. A., Pedersen, N. L., Fratiglioni, L., . . . Gatz, M. (2012). Work-related stress may increase the risk of vascular dementia. *Journal of the American Geriatrics Society, 60*(1), 60-67.

Andel, R., Crowe, M., Kareholt, I., Wastesson, J., & Parker, M. G. (2011). Indicators of job strain at midlife and cognitive functioning in advanced old age. *Journals of Gerontology Series B: Psychological Sciences and Social Sciences, 66*(3), 287-291.

Andel, R., Crowe, M., Pedersen, N. L., Mortimer, J., Crimmins, E., Johansson, B., & Gatz, M. (2005). Complexity of work and risk of Alzheimer's disease: A population-based study of Swedish twins. *Journals of Gerontolology Series B: Psychological Sciences and Social Sciences, 60*(5), P251-258.

Andel, R., Hughes, T. F., & Crowe, M. (2005). Strategies to reduce the risk of cognitive decline and dementia. *Aging Health, 1*(1), 107-116.

Andel, R., Kareholt, I., Parker, M. G., Thorslund, M., & Gatz, M. (2007). Complexity of primary lifetime occupation and cognition in advanced old age. *Journal of Aging and Health, 19*(3), 397-415.

Andel, R., Vigen, C., Mack, W. J., Clark, L. J., & Gatz, M. (2006). The effect of education and occupational complexity on rate of cognitive decline in Alzheimer's patients. *Journal of the International Neuropsychological Society, 12*(1), 147-152.

Anttila, T., Helkala, E. L., Kivipelto, M., Hallikainen, M., Alhainen, K., Heinonen, H., . . . Nissinen, A. (2002). Midlife income, occupation, APOE status, and dementia: A population-based study. *Neurology, 59*(6), 887-893.

Ashford, J. W., & Mortimer, J. A. (2002). Non-familial Alzheimer's disease is mainly due to genetic factors. *Journal of Alzheimer's Disease, 4*(3), 169-177.

Azzimondi, G., D'Alessandro, R., Pandolfo, G., & Feruglio, F. S. (1998). Comparative study of the prevalence of dementia in two Sicilian communities with different psychological backgrounds. *Neuroepidemiology, 17,* 199-209.

Belkic, K. L., Landsbergis, P. A., Schnall, P. L., & Baker, D. (2004). Is job strain a major source of cardiovascular disease risk? *Scandinavian Journal of Work, Environment & Health, 30*(2), 85-128.

Calvo, E., Sarkisian N., & Tamborini C. R. (2013). Causal effects of retirement timing on subjective physical and emotional health. *J Gerontol B Psychol Sci Soc Sci, 68*(1), 73-84.

Canadian Study of Health and Aging. (1994). The Canadian Study of Health and Aging: Risk factors for Alzheimer's disease in Canada. *Neurology, 44,* 2073–2080.

Coe, N. B., von Gaudecker, H. M., Lindeboom, M., & Maurer, J. (2012). The effect of retirement on cognitive functioning. *Health Economics, 21*(8), 913-927.

Crowe, M., Andel, R., Pedersen, N. L., Fratiglioni, L., & Gatz, M. (2006). Personality and risk of cognitive impairment 25 years later. *Psychology and Aging, 21*(3), 573-580.

Crowe, M., Andel, R., Pedersen, N. L., & Gatz, M. (2007). Do work-related stress and reactivity to stress predict dementia more than 30 years later? *Alzheimer Disease & Associated Disorders, 21*(3), 205-209.

Ekerdt, D. J., Kosloski, K., & DeViney, S. (2000). The normative anticipation of retirement by older workers. *Research on Aging, 22*(1), 3-22.

Eller, N. H., Netterstrom, B., Gyntelberg, F., Kristensen, T. S., Nielsen, F., Steptoe, A., & Theorell, T. (2009). Work-related psychosocial factors and the development of ischemic heart disease: A systematic review. *Cardiology in Review, 17*(2), 83-97.

Evans, D. A., Hebert, L. E., Beckett, L. A., Scherr, P. A., Albert, M. S., Chown, M. J., . . . Schaie K. W. (1997). Education and other measures of socioeconomic status and risk of incident Alzheimer disease in a defined population of older persons. *Archives of Neurology, 54,* 1399-1405.

Finch, C. E., & Seeman, T. E. (1999). Stress theories of aging. In V. L. Bengston & K. W. Schaie (Eds.), *Handbook of theories of aging* (pp. 81-97). New York, NY: Springer Publishing Company, Inc.

Finkel, D., Andel, R., Gatz, M., & Pedersen, N. L. (2009). The role of occupational complexity in trajectories of cognitive aging before and after retirement. *Psychology and Aging, 24*(3), 563-573.

Finkel, D., Reynolds, C. A., McArdle, J. J., & Pedersen, N. L. (2005). The longitudinal relationship between processing speed and cognitive ability: Genetic and environmental influences. *Behavior Genetics, 35*(5), 535-549.

Forstmeier, S., Maercker, A., Maier, W., van den Bussche, H., Riedel-Heller, S., Kaduszkiewicz, H., . . . Wagner, M. (2012). Motivational reserve: Motivation-related occupational abilities and risk of mild cognitive impairment and Alzheimer disease. *Psychology and Aging, 27*(2), 353-363.

Gatz, M. (2005). Educating the brain to avoid dementia: Can mental exercise prevent Alzheimer disease? *PLoS Med, 2*(1), e7.

Gatz, M., Svedberg, P., Pedersen, N. L., Mortimer, J. A., Berg, S., & Johansson, B. (2001). Education and the risk of Alzheimer's Disease: Findings from the Study of Dementia in Swedish Twins. *Journals of Gerontology: Psychological Sciences, 56B,* P292–P300.

Heckhausen, J., Wrosch, C., & Schulz, R. (2010). A motivational theory of life-span development. *Psychological Review, 117*(1), 32.

Heeringa, S. G., & Connor, J. (1995). Technical description of the Health and Retirement Study Sample Design. http://hrsonline.isr.umich.edu/sitedocs/userg/HRSSAMP.pdf.

Helman, R., Greenwald, M., VanDerhei, J., & Copeland, C. (2007). Minority workers remain confident about retirement, despite lagging preparations and false expectations. *EBRI Issue Brief, 306,* 1-18.

Helmer, C., Letenneur, L., Rouch, I., Richard-Harston, S., Barberger-Gateau, P., Fabrigoule, C., . . . Dartigues, J. F. (2001). Occupation during life and risk of dementia in French elderly community residents. *Journal of Neurology, Neurosurgery & Psychiatry, 71*, 303-309.

Hughes, T. F., & Ganguli, M. (2009). Modifiable midlife risk factors for late-life cognitive impairment and dementia. *Current Psychiatry Reviews, 5*(2), 73-92.

Kaplan, G. A., Turrell, G., Lynch, J. W., Everson, S. A., Helkala, E. L., & Salonen, J. T. (2001). Childhood socioeconomic position and cognitive function in adulthood. *International Journal of Epidemiology, 30*, 256-263.

Karasek, R. (1979). Job demands, job decision, latitude, and mental strain: Implications for job redesign. *Administrative Science Quarterly 24*, 285-308.

Karasek, R., & Theorell, T. (1990). *Healthy work: Stress, productivity, and the reconstruction of working life.* New York: Basic Books.

Karp, A., Andel, R., Parker, M. G., Wang, H. X., Winblad, B., & Fratiglioni, L. (2009). Mentally stimulating activities at work during midlife and dementia risk after age 75: Follow-up study from the Kungsholmen Project. *American Journal of Geriatric Psychiatry, 17*(3), 227-236.

Kiecolt-Glaser, J. K., McGuire, L., Robles, T. F., & Glaser, R. (2002). Psychoneuroimmunology and psychosomatic medicine: Back to the future. *Psychosomatic Medicine, 64*, 15-28.

Kim, J. E., & Moen, P. (2002). Retirement transitions, gender, and psychological well-being a life-course, ecological model. *The Journals of Gerontology Series B: Psychological Sciences and Social Sciences, 57*(3), P212-P222.

Kohn, M. L., & Schooler, C. (1983). *Work and personality: An inquiry into the impact of social stratification.* Norwood, NJ: Ablex.

Kroger, E., Andel, R., Lindsay, J., Benounissa, Z., Verreault, R., & Laurin, D. (2008). Is complexity of work associated with risk of dementia? The Canadian Study of Health and Aging. *American Journal of Epidemiology, 167*(7), 820-830.

Launer, L. J. (2002). Demonstrating the case that AD is a vascular disease: Epidemiologic evidence. *Ageing Research Reviews, 1*(1), 61-77.

McEwen, B. S. (1998). Stress, adaptation, and disease. Allostasis and allostatic load. *Annals of the New York Academy of Sciences, 840*, 33-44.

McEwen, B. S. (2007). Physiology and neurobiology of stress and adaptation: Central role of the brain. [Review]. *Physiological Reviews, 87*(3), 873-904.

McFall, B. H. (2011). Crash and wait? The impact of the Great Recession on retirement planning of older Americans. *American Economic Review, 101*(3), 40-44.

Mermin, G. B., Johnson, R. W., & Murphy, D. P. (2007). Why do boomers plan to work longer? *Journals of Gerontolology Series B: Psychological Sciences and Social Sciences, 62*(5), S286-S294.

Moceri, V. M., Kukull, W. A., Emanuel, I., van Belle, G., & Larson, E. B. (2000). Early-life risk factors and the development of Alzheimer's disease. *Neurology, 54*(2), 415-420.

Ngandu, T., von Strauss, E., Helkala, E. L., Winblad, B., Nissinen, A., Tuomilehto, J., . . . Kivipelto, M. (2007). Education and dementia: What lies behind the association? *Neurology, 69*(14), 1442-1450.

Paykel, E. S., Brayne, C., Huppert, F. A., Gill, C., Barkley, C., Gehlhaar, E., . . . O'Connor, D. (1994). Incidence of dementia in a population older than 75 years in the United Kingdom. *Archives of General Psychiatry, 51*, 325–332.

Plomin, R. (1999). Genetics and general cognitive ability. *Nature, 402*(6761 Suppl), C25-C29.

Poirier, J. (2000). Apolipoprotein E and Alzheimer's disease. A role in amyloid catabolism. *Annals of the New York Academy of Sciences, 924*, 81-90.

Potter, G. G., Helms, M. J., Burke, J. R., Steffens, D. C., & Plassman, B. L. (2007). Job demands and dementia risk among male twin pairs. *Alzheimer's and Dementia, 3*(3), 192-199.

Potter, G. G., Plassman, B. L., Helms, M. J., Foster, S. M., & Edwards, N. W. (2006). Occupational characteristics and cognitive performance among elderly male twins. *Neurology, 67*(8), 1377-1382.

Qui, C., Karp, A., von Strauss, E., Winblad, B., Fratiglioni, L., & Bellander, T. (2003). Lifetime principal occupation and risk of Alzheimer's disease in the Kungsholmen project. *American Journal of Industrial Medicine, 43*, 204-211.

Ravaglia, G., Forti, P., Maioli, F., Sacchetti, L., Mariani, E., Nativio, V., . . . Macini, P. L. (2002). Education, occupation, and prevalence of dementia: Findings from the Conselice Study. *Dementia and Geriatric Cognitive Disorders, 14*, 90-100.

Ravona-Springer, R., Beeri, M. S., & Goldbourt, U. (2013). Satisfaction with current status at work and lack of motivation to improve it during midlife is associated with increased risk for dementia in subjects who survived thirty-seven years later. *Journal of Alzheimer's Disease, 36*(4), 769-80.

Rohwedder, S., & Willis, R. J. (2010). Mental retirement. *Journal of Economic Perspectives, 24*(1), 119-138.

Salthouse, T. A. (2006). Mental exercise and mental aging evaluating the validity of the "use it or lose it" hypothesis. *Perspectives on Psychological Science, 1*(1), 68-87.

Salthouse, T. A. (2009). When does age-related cognitive decline begin? *Neurobiology of Aging, 30*(4), 507-514.

Sapolsky, R. M. (1996). Why stress is bad for your brain. *Science, 273*, 749-750.

Schaie, K. W. (2005). *Development influences on adult intelligence: The Seattle Longitudinal Study.* New York: Oxford University Press.

Schooler, C. (1984). Psychological effects of complex environment during the life span: A review and theory. *Intelligence, 8,* 259-281.

Schooler, C., Mulatu, M. S., & Oates, G. (1999). The continuing effects of substantively complex work on the intellectual functioning of older workers. *Psychology and Aging, 14,* 483-506.

Seidler, A., Nienhaus, A., Bernhardt, T., Kauppinen, T., Elo, A. L., & Frolich, L. (2004). Psychosocial work factors and dementia. *Occupational and Environmental Medicine, 61*(12), 962-971.

Sharp, E. S., & Gatz, M. (2011). Relationship between education and dementia: An updated systematic review. *Alzheimer Disease & Associated Disorders, 25*(4), 289-304.

Stern, Y. (2002). What is cognitive reserve? Theory and research application of the reserve concept. *Journal of the International Neuropsychological Society, 8*(3), 448-460.

Stern, Y. (2012). Cognitive reserve in ageing and Alzheimer's disease. *The Lancet Neurolology, 11*(11), 1006-1012.

Stern, Y., Alexander, G. E., Prohovnik, I., Stricks, L., Link, B., Lennon, M. C., Mayeux, R. (1995). Relationship between lifetime occupation and parietal flow: Implications for a reserve against Alzheimer's disease pathology. *Neurology, 45,* 55-60.

Stern, Y., Gurland, B., Tatemichi, T. K., Tang, M. X., Wilder, D., & Mayeux, R. (1994). Influence of education and occupation on the incidence of Alzheimer's disease. *Journal of the American Medical Association, 271,* 1004–1010.

Szinovacz, M. E., Martin L., & Davey A. (2014). Recession and Expected Retirement Age: Another Look at the Evidence. *Gerontologist, 54*(2), 245-257.

U.S. Department of Labor. (1977). *Dictionary of occupational titles* (4th ed.). Washington, DC: U.S. Government Printing Office.

Voorhees, R. (2001). *Old age is always 15 years older than I am.* Kansas City, MI: Andrews McMeel Publishing.

Wang, H. X., Karp, A., Herlitz, A., Crowe, M., Kareholt, I., Winblad, B., & Fratiglioni, L. (2009). Personality and lifestyle in relation to dementia incidence. *Neurology, 72*(3), 253-259.

Wang, H. X., Wahlberg, M., Karp, A., Winblad, B., & Fratiglioni, L. (2012). Psychosocial stress at work is associated with increased dementia risk in late life. *Alzheimers & Dementia, 8*(2), 114-120.

Weinstein, G., Wolf, P. A., Beiser, A. S., Au, R., & Seshadri, S. (2013). Risk estimations, risk factors, and genetic variants associated with Alzheimer's disease in selected publications from the Framingham Heart Study. *Journal of Alzheimer's Disease, 33 Suppl 1,* S439-S445.

Wilson, R. S., Scherr, P. A., Hoganson, G., Bienias, J. L., Evans, D. A., & Bennett, D. A. (2005). Early life socioeconomic status and late life risk of Alzheimer's disease. *Neuroepidemiology, 25*(1), 8-14.

Yaffe, K., Vittinghoff, E., Lindquist, K., Barnes, D., Covinsky, K. E., Neylan, T., . . . Marmar, C. (2010). Posttraumatic stress disorder and risk of dementia among US veterans. *Archives of General Psychiatry, 67*(6), 608-613.

Volunteering

Caroline Wolverson, DipCOT, DipHT, MSc

This is the real secret of life—to be completely engaged with what you are doing in the here and now. And instead of calling it work, realize it is play.—Alan Watts (1977)

In the current socioeconomic climate, there is an increasing requirement for volunteers to support services in meeting the health and social care needs of communities. The importance of maintaining the social and economic contribution of older people within society has been recognized for some time by policy makers. It could be argued that older people are ideally placed to make up a major component of the voluntary sector following retirement; not only to assist them in maintaining a productive lifestyle that contributes to their health and well-being, but enabling them to continue to contribute to society. The concept of productive aging recognizes the knowledge, experience, and skills that older people can offer, and volunteering gives society the opportunity to utilize these (Morrow-Howell, Carden, & Sherraden, 2005). Van Dyne and Farmer (2005) suggest that volunteering can become not just what a person does, but who they are, which contributes to a positive sense of role identity (see Chapter 2).

The contribution of older people to the volunteer sector is significant; 24% of people over 65 in the United States have done some form of volunteering in the past year (U.S. Department of Labor, 2011), with 44.9% of these volunteering for religious organizations. A major policy agenda of the Obama administration has been promotion of volunteering with a program specifically designed to recruit older people (Tang, 2010).

Volunteering can take many forms, from supporting family and friends to being involved with formal organizations. For the purposes of this chapter, it will be defined as "any activity in which time is given freely to benefit another person, group, or organization" (Wilson, 2000, p. 215). This chapter will consider the benefits, challenges, and motivations for volunteering. It will highlight difficulties of recruiting and maintaining older volunteers and how systems can support this group of people who may have a range of health and social care needs themselves. Six people between the ages of 65 and 81 told their stories for this chapter; these will be used to illustrate findings from research.

Hunt LA, Wolverson C.
Work and the Older Person: Increasing Longevity and Well-Being (pp 101-111).
© 2015 SLACK Incorporated.

BENEFITS TO THE PERSON

Warburton, Paynter, and Petriwskyj (2007) identified volunteering as a key dimension of both healthy and productive ageing. Volunteering can offer the opportunity for continued personal development and lifelong learning as identified in a study by Lie, Baines, and Wheelock (2009), which highlighted the opportunity it brings for choice, freedom, and flexibility. In addition, Warburton (2006) suggests that the role of volunteer can help to build self-esteem and give a sense of control; all of which may contribute to positive feelings of self-worth and a sense of well-being. Lum & Lightfoot (2005) confirmed previous studies that found that those who volunteer show less decline in self-reported health and functioning levels.

When asked if they felt volunteering contributed to their health, June (73) and Barbara (81) both responded positively:

> *Barbara: You hear other people's troubles and you go home and think how lucky you are and count your blessings. You see people like a couple of my friends who spend their time sleeping. Well, I could be like that but I know I feel better getting washed and dressed and the routine I get.*
>
> *June: It gets us up in the morning, out and meeting folk. You see, I think if you are poorly and can't raise yourself to get out amongst people, you sit at home and think I'm poorly… I'm poorly; you stay in the four walls and you do feel poorly, and then if you stay in the next day and stay in bed as well—oh I can't stay in bed.*

There is still, to some degree, an ageist view that older people are largely consumers of health and social care resources, without considering their contributions to maintaining a functioning society. This view could have a detrimental effect on an individual's feelings of self-worth; however, this negative attitude may be reinforced by older people themselves, as was highlighted by Catherine (66), a retired university lecturer, when asked if she felt that society was limiting her opportunities or making assumptions about her since she retired:

> *I think it's me that's making assumptions. I haven't had any evidence in my own life… except, there is this woman in my supermarket that refers to me very patronizingly every time she serves me as "darling" and it drives me crackers. I take it that it's because I'm 66, but she does it to everyone I'm sure. But no, I actually haven't had any impact from society, I think it's my own attitude. Good grief, I'm getting old, I'm nearer 70 now than I am 60!*

The maintenance of physical health not only contributes to the well-being of older people, but enables them to continue to contribute to society. Interestingly, for those interviewed, the physical health benefits to volunteering were not just identified in the volunteering acts themselves, but from getting to the location. This was raised by Mike (78), a retired shipping agent who visits the sick in the parish:

> *I suppose it has an effect on my health because it gets me out. I walk to the visits I do for the Society of St. Vincent de Paul. When I volunteered at the hospital, you could claim petrol money, but I didn't. I would try to go on my bike but it was hard work!*

Likewise, Ray (80), a retired electrician, maintains his physical fitness by cycling to his volunteer work, as pointed out by his wife:

> *June:…and you don't realize, Ray only has a push bike to get him to the scout hut 2 miles away; it's held together with rust and paint!*
>
> *Ray: Oh yes, it keeps me fit, I enjoy doing it. I've got a bit of arthritis in my knee and it gives me trouble at times but you can't stop, you've got to keep going. It gets you up and wears you out. I think when you're retired you've got to keep going, it doesn't matter what, you've got to keep going and get on with things.*

Socialization can contribute to continued health and well-being for older people. This age group is more vulnerable to social isolation for a number of reasons: loss of physical function, loss of confidence, and gradual loss of friends and family (University of Brighton, Age UK Brighton, Hove & Portslade, 2012). A study of women volunteers by Parkinson, Warburton, Sibbritt, and Byles (2010) found that they reported a higher quality of life and social support than those who did not volunteer. Speaking of her volunteering at the church shop, Barbara stated:

> And we like to find out all the gossip. We have a coffee break at 11 sharp and about 10 of us sit in a circle and out it all comes; ailments, places we've been, June always mentions her rambling, which is interesting. And there's laughter and jokes, and we get first look at the clothes and books and try things on.

MOTIVATION TO VOLUNTEER

Altruism is often a major motivating factor in volunteering. A study by Morrow-Howell, Hong, and Tang (2009) confirmed earlier research identifying that contribution to others and the community, along with making a difference to people's lives, were the most widely reported benefits. The study also recognized the large number of participants who felt their lives were improved as a result of volunteering, and it was suggested that this might be associated with increased self-esteem, increased self-efficacy, and increased socialization. This was confirmed by Lie, Baines, and Wheelock (2009), who highlighted how volunteers valued volunteering as a source of happiness and joy, giving them the "feel good" (p. 709) factor.

Altruism is again referred to in a study by Cook (2011) that focuses on the Women's Royal Voluntary Service (WRVS), who have 45,000 volunteers throughout Great Britain. In her interview with John, who cared for his wife, he spoke of the desire to "give something back" (p. 143). Having experienced the benefit of care services for his wife, he now works as a volunteer driver.

The motivation offered through faith is shown by the number of volunteers linked to religious organizations. All six people interviewed for this chapter are involved in volunteering activities linked to the church, with two of those specifically referring to their faith as a motivating factor. Mike (78) has volunteered in a variety of roles since the age of 24. He states one of his reasons for volunteering:

> Well I suppose because I'm a Christian I think you should be doing something for your fellow man. I suppose I get a sense of satisfaction; the fella who still lives at home that I visit every week is very appreciative. The knowledge that it's needed motivates me to volunteer.

Catherine, who now spends much of her time volunteering both through the church and the university where she was previously employed, explains her motivation:

> Well, that's the thing; I've got the skills, many thanks to God. I mean he is key, Number 1 in what I do because every January, I sit down with what I'm doing and pray it all through. I've been given abilities and skills and don't think it's right to keep them to myself if I'm still able to use them, which I suppose might sound a bit big-headed, but that's not what I mean.

Recognition of commitment to volunteering can also bring its own rewards. Jean Bishop (90) has been fundraising for Age Concern for the past 30 years. She is known locally as the "bee lady" because she dresses as a bumblebee and collects money. She was rewarded in the summer of 2012 by being nominated to carry the Olympic Torch. The publicity she received from this has increased her donations, which to-date stand at £87,000. Her aim is to reach £100,000. She states: "There is no such thing as retiring. Once I reach the target, I'll start again." In addition to her fundraising, Jean also organizes a "knit and natter" for older women each week (Longhorn, 2012).

Interestingly, in studies by Finkelstein (2008) and Penner, Dovidio, Pilavin, and Schroeder (2005), findings showed that initially, volunteering met an altruistic need. However, as time progressed, outcomes were more focused on personal development. Rochester and Hutchison with Harris and Keely (2002) also found important personal motivators to keep active and involved, feel useful, meet new people, and provide routine. Another positive outcome of the volunteering role is that the personal development it offers may bring opportunity for future paid employment. This was referred to by Rachel (65), who carries out a number of voluntary roles in an advisory capacity to a range of health and social care organizations:

> *Well, I wouldn't have applied for the jobs in the Department of Health if I hadn't done the volunteering because I wouldn't have known about them. I came to them laterally; I wasn't sort of sitting in some isolated provincial place, looking at the hallowed halls, thinking oh, I'll have a go at that. Because I've got a perception working [there], I knew something about the characters, personalities, and mechanisms, both overt and covert. It had certain attractions for me because I felt if I could fit in there. I knew enough to exert some leverage from the word go, and because it was a 3-day-a-week post, it would still give me the opportunity to do other things.*

Routine was a significant factor referred to by those who told their stories. Lack of routine following retirement can have a detrimental effect on an individual's health. The development of new routines can be challenging. Davis Smith and Gay (2005) found the most commonly reported age-related incentives for volunteering were to fill the gap left by work following retirement, and manage the increased time available. This was referred to by Mike, who retired from full-time work at the age of 60.

> *About 6 months after I retired, I was so fed up of doing nothing that I went to work as a volunteer at the local hospital. They were asking for volunteers and I worked on two wards. I would go in about 9:30 in the morning, make the tea and serve it, then collect and wash the empties. Then later on I would go out with the dinner plates. I did it for about 2 years.*

Ray (80) and June (73) have been married for 50 years. Both retired at 58. Ray was an electrician with his own business. June had done the accounting for Ray's business and brought up two children, then opened a clothes shop about 10 years before she retired. They have done some form of volunteering throughout their lives, but their volunteer work has increased since retirement.

> **June:** *After the last grandchild went to school, I started with the church shop. I went to the person that manages the shop and asked if I could help. She said there Mondays & Tuesdays were available and I said I would do both, and she said, "Oh we don't normally get people volunteering for 2 days!" Working at the church, it gets me up in the morning. You need a routine as you get older.*
>
> **Ray:** *Well this was the thing. Monday and Tuesday it was church volunteering, Wednesday there was going to the supermarket on the free bus. Thursday was helping at the school, and Friday was our free day, but that's changed now because June volunteers at the museum, so we don't have a free day really.*

June and her friend of nearly 50 years, Barbara, refer to the importance of routine in their lives:

> **Barbara:** *You need a routine as you get older.*
>
> **June:** *I agree. I'm really happy, I love getting up and thinking I'm doing this today, I'm doing that today. There's a lot of people who just sit there not doing anything, and they could and would feel a lot better I'm sure, but then everybody's different.*
>
> **Barbara:** *Working at the church—it gets us up in the morning.*
>
> **Ray:** *The main thing is waking up in the morning!*
>
> **Barbara:** *I get my clothes ready the night before in case I can't do it in the morning. Sometimes I think, oh heck! Will I be able to manage? But then when I get there, I can, and it's fine.*

In speaking of his work with the Scouts and maintaining the Scout hut, Ray referred to both a sense of responsibility and the feeling of a job well done:

Ray: Well, they leave me alone for one thing; they just say, "Do whatever you think needs doing," but no one else wants to do it. There was one chap before me, he used to come down on the bus and clean, but he's gone now.

June: And when they haven't got Ray, there's no one else!

Ray: They used to call me to say this light's gone or that door's damaged, and it was pathetic some of the repairs that were done. The maintenance got really bad, the toilets were terrible, so I tiled the two bathroom floors and fitted hot water to one of the toilets. I get the satisfaction of sorting things out.

June: He likes doing things right.

For those telling their stories, there are several motivating factors—routine, altruism, satisfaction from a job well done, and faith—that all contributed to continued well-being for those involved.

Informal Volunteering—Caring for Family and Friends

Informal caregivers are often vulnerable to poor health themselves; however, this form of volunteering can bring many rewards. Cook (2011) notes that 65% of older people regularly help older neighbors. Barbara (81) has lived in the same house since 1960 and has had some of the same neighbors for all of this time. This aging community supports each other well. Barbara was a constant support to her good friend and neighbor Eve as her health deteriorated, supplementing the care provided by Eve's son and professional services. When asked why she took on this caring role, she responded:

Because Eve had a bachelor son, and he had nobody else to help him. She said specifically that she wanted to die in her own home, so I went and sat [with her] while he went to the gym to get a break, and it just went on like that. I sat by the bed. It was hard work and I was frightened half the time [because] I was on my own at night with her often. Then the caregiver used to come at about 10 pm to stay overnight until 6 am.

I can't say no. I suppose it's not the thing to do. It's how you're brought up. Besides, how could you leave a man like that? He was hopeless; he was hysterical if he saw a spider, even at the age of 50! And Eve knew he was helpless, she left me a small amount of money and I know it was because she knew I would help. I mean, I wouldn't have done it for money, of course, but I knew that was why she did it. And then afterwards, helping him to clear out the house took a long time, there was so much stuff.

I didn't get anything from doing it, I don't think, but she had been my friend for nearly 50 years and I admired her. She was interesting and she was generous with rides in the car. She said things that other people wanted to and didn't, and she was disliked by quite a few people for that, but she was a good friend.

Barbara also spoke of the way that caring roles "happen," rather than being planned or by choice:

My mother came to live with me when I was about 66. She was here for nearly 5 years, and before that, she and Dad had lived with my brother and his wife for about 15 years. Things happen without anyone asking you to do it. You are there, and without you knowing or being asked, it happens. My brother didn't ask for Mother to move to live with me, it just seemed to happen. Mother once said to me, "You took me in when no one else would have me." But it just went along like that. My sister-in-law became more ill and I used to go down to stay and help about four times a year, and I really worked when I was there, but it was family and it was no hardship. I was with family and it was OK. But nobody said, "Would you do this?" I was just there and no one else was there. I liked having Mother here with me.

This role has also happened to Barbara with two of her long-time friends:

I have two friends and these days I don't have the friendship that I used to have with them. There is no conversation, they don't remember what I've said [about] making appointments to meet or go places. I have to keep tabs on them. Kate calls me and she's lost £50 here and there and she hasn't really, she's just hidden it between towels or pockets of different coats or behind the telephone rack. I remember the places she's hidden it before and I say, how about looking there or there. I get phone calls telling me about things that have happened again and again. So my friendships aren't what they used to be; there's no support for me there anymore.

Grandparents have taken on an increasingly important role in sustaining both the family and society as unpaid caregivers of grandchildren. A study by Pepin and Deutscher (2011) found that the role of grandparent was particularly meaningful to the participants and accounted for a significant amount of their time. A recent article by Uglow (2012) interviewed a number of grandparents. Their reasons for the high level of childcare they provided include not wanting to be a distant grandparent, supporting their children in giving them a bit of a break, and being part of a young family. Another reason noted was that this generation of grandparents are the Baby Boomers who were focused on their careers and missed out on time with their own children, so they are making up for it now.

Although informal volunteering can bring its rewards, it can also be detrimental to health. Barbara spoke of a time 10 years ago when she was not only caring for her mother, but also providing support to two neighbors:

I know it's an old-fashioned term, but I'm sure I had a nervous breakdown toward the end of mum's life. It happened when I was in church. It was the end of the service and I felt really ill. It passed, but that was the start of it. I'm talking about 10 years ago, but I still have feelings about that mentally I think. My daughter got me a very good book to read and when I felt these feelings of anxiety coming on, I flew to this book and sat quietly and read it over and over again and that helped me no end. I still have that book.

I never thought about it being due to having too much to do and not being able to keep up my own routines, but looking back, that was perhaps what started it. I still have guilt regarding putting Mother in a nursing home because I now realize I could have had more help if I had gone about it in the right way. That guilt is with me all the time.

When I had my mother here, I was also supporting two other neighbors. Anita had rheumatoid arthritis; I used to shop for her and make her tea. I'd go over and get her up if she'd had a fall. But now the National Health Service is marvelous. With Anne (another neighbor of 90), I don't go there every day like I used to; the doctor told me to back off! She gets home care visits 3 times a day now, and that seems to be working well. It was almost a full-time job at one point with Mother and two neighbors, but it's just helping people isn't it? People do that all the time. I hardly go to Anne's now. I go on Wednesdays because I empty the rubbish bins and put them out. People give her flowers, so I tend to those, but I don't do anything else now. Oh, and I also go next door to Bob's to let the dog out at lunchtime, but that doesn't take long.

There are many positive benefits to informal caregiving, but the need to support those who volunteer in this way must be addressed to ensure they maintain their own good health. For many, like Barbara, there is often no choice but to take on this role, and although it may be satisfying, it can also become overwhelming. Informal caregivers need to be aware of support that is available to them, and should be encouraged to take advantage of it.

BENEFITS TO THE COMMUNITY

The importance of those working in the nonprofit sector to the makeup of society's complex social systems is highlighted by Warburton and Jeppsson Grassman (2009). Volunteering represents a critical component of how societies are organized (Anheier & Salamon, 1999). A study by the WRVS (2011) estimated that those over age 65 made a net contribution of £40 billion (approximately 59 billion U.S. dollars) to the UK economy in 2010; a significant proportion of this was through the provision of social care and the value of volunteering. In considering globalization and citizenship, volunteering offers potential for diverse populations to be integrated, enhancing social capital and assisting in maintaining a democratic society (Putnam, 2000). Tang (2010) highlights the importance of strategies to encourage engagement of older people, particularly those from disadvantaged groups, in volunteering. This would not only encourage a more integrated society, but also potentially improve the health and well-being of disadvantaged and marginalized groups.

Those interviewed spoke of the community benefits of their volunteer work. Barbara helps out for 2 hours a week sorting donations for the weekly sale at the village church; she then attends the sale, where cooked meals are provided by other volunteers (including June) for the community at low cost. The weekly event raises money for the maintenance of the church, but also provides an opportunity for a hot meal and social contact.

> **Barbara:** *I joined [as a church volunteer] because I've lived [here] for 50 years and in some small way I wanted to give something back, and June of course introduced me to it.*
>
> **June:** *On Fridays I work in the school museum; the work is enjoyable. I was in on the first day it opened. It was the oldest school in the area and the council wanted to knock it down and make it into a car park, so the vicar objected. They said we could keep it if we used it for educational purposes.*
>
> *We have a liaison who coordinates local schools coming in, and there was all this stuff from the school that was still there, and all the photographs. We decided to keep it all and set up the museum. Anyone that came would say things like, "Would you like this, it was my mother's, etc." We are just cataloging it all.*
>
> **Barbara:** *I was so pleased that the cradle I gave was still there; Mrs. Clapman gave me that when I was a child and she was about 90, and it's still there on display with a doll in it.*
>
> **June:** *Yes, and the shawl on the doll was made by my grandmother. She lived to be 92 and couldn't see all that well, but she still crocheted all the time.*
>
> *They decided we would open the museum for 4 hours a week. We are getting people from far and wide, and they write nice comments, saying how friendly or helpful we are. People doing their family history come week after week and use the computer. It's mainly talking to people; lovely listening to people's background stories. You do have a laugh really.*

These shared experiences offer an opportunity for social connectedness, giving volunteers a sense of belonging, which Warburton and Jeppsson Grassman (2009) highlight as significant to health and well-being.

CHALLENGES TO RECRUITING AND SUSTAINING VOLUNTEERS

Rochester and Hitchison with Harris and Keely (2002) found several barriers to volunteering. Some organizations had restrictions such as age limits on volunteers and fewer roles for older volunteers. A second barrier highlighted by the World Health Organization (WHO, 2007) and Gill (2006) was attitudes of older people themselves, such as not knowing what volunteering entailed and lack of confidence. Further barriers were practical issues such as poverty, restricted mobility, transport, and finance. The final area identified was cultural barriers, such as some cultures not having a tradition of volunteering, or language barriers that may occur. Although Mike (78) still volunteers, he spoke of the physical limitations that affecting his volunteering:

> *I volunteered every year taking sick people on the church visit to Lourdes until I got too old to do it; I stopped 5 or 6 years ago because I was no longer physically able. When I first went, we were on duty from about 6 in the morning. We would have to get the men out of bed, get them dressed and fed, then we had to pull them around during the day. Now I just go there for a holiday each year. I'm still on the Lourdes sick fund committee and we meet about 4 times a year. I was treasurer for about 15 years and a member of the committee as well. I had to go up to Middlesbrough 4 times a year, which was about a 6-hour trip. I'm not as alert as I used to be, that's why I gave up driving, so that has changed the things I volunteer for. I used to drive older people to a weekly church group and can't do this anymore either.*

Physical limitations that often come with advancing age should not exclude older people from volunteering; rather, attempts should be made to encourage continued engagement through different means.

Over recent years, there has been an increased professionalization and formalization of volunteering as identified by Lie, Baines, and Wheelock (2009). A potential danger is that this may give rise to a reluctance to volunteer for those who do not want too great a commitment. In addition, existing volunteers who find that their roles are becoming more demanding may feel increased pressure, which can have a detrimental effect on their well-being.

The WHO (2007) recognizes the need for volunteers to receive adequate training. In their report, older people state that opportunities for volunteering and employment should be tailored to the person's needs and interests. For example, just because an individual has a disability and receives services, this should not exclude him or her from offering a service to others. A study for the WRVS (Cook, 2011) commented on the recruitment of volunteers from those who had received services. They offer a short-term support service on hospital discharge, and have found that those who receive a service often want to become involved in providing this service once they are well again.

The limitations of the person should be recognized, and job matching should be considered, just as it would be in mainstream employment. This was something that was identified by June (73), who has volunteered for several years in different roles at the weekly church sale and lunch.

> *When I first started, I was put on furniture and that was difficult. I was assessing how much to charge, and there was a delivery lad who I knew wasn't being honest, but how do you explain that to the church people? It made it quite difficult. Anyway, I said I wanted to get out of the furniture, and he left around the same time, but there were more rules and regulations for furniture and electrical, so they scrapped all that. I was put in the kitchen, where I said I would never ever go, but all I do is wash dishes and clean tables. There is no pressure on me whatsoever, and so I'm happy cleaning up, which I never thought I would be. The only thing is, after the meals I have to lug all the tables and I'm finding that a bit hard. Everyone is conscious that if you don't do it, no one else will. It's a responsibility; you can't get the volunteers. Quite a few start and then you don't see them again. When this group leaves, I don't think it will continue. It's been going for 30 years. There is one person a bit younger than me. There are about four in their 80s. I do feel a sense of responsibility to keep doing it.*

The location of the volunteer work is particularly important to older people. A number of studies identified travel as a factor in volunteering (Cook, 2011; WHO, 2007), as well as reimbursement for travel expenses.

Others plan their daily lives around their volunteering activities, as Catherine points out:

> *…And I made sure that when I moved, I could cut straight through to the hospital, church, and university, so I could still walk to all of them, but now I'm ground floor rather than second floor.*

The range of barriers presented to older people are not insurmountable; however, society must address these real concerns and provide necessary support systems to encourage continued volunteering by older people, and encourage older people to see volunteering as a positive option in maintaining their health and well-being.

SUPPORTING VOLUNTEERS

In her study of the WRVS, Cook (2011) gave several recommendations for organizations to support and encourage those who volunteer: clear roles, using existing skills and developing new ones, training, and support. In addition, consideration should be given to flexibility, and recognizing that the person may not want to do the same thing over many years (Ford, 2008).

Although there are many volunteers working in charities and the private sector, volunteering is not as frequently seen in the public sector. The UK government's focus on partnership across organizations (public, private, and voluntary sectors) offers the opportunity for knowledge sharing by the voluntary sector, which enables the public sector to use volunteers effectively (Preedy, 2012). Volunteering should not be viewed as static; volunteers should be offered the opportunity for personal development and given a clear role. Commitment to maintaining and sustaining volunteers within an organization is required, with clearly identified roles that will assist the organization and the volunteer. Clear standards should be identified, such as those provided by Investing in Volunteers (United Kingdom Voluntary Forum, 2012), the UK standard that provides quality accreditation to organizations that have a volunteer workforce.

Tang, Morrow-Howell, and Hong (2007) found that strategies such as choice and enabling volunteers to set their own schedule can assist in making volunteer work attractive to older people, as noted by Ray:

> *…some of the jobs, I can think, oh I don't need to do that today; I can sweep the yard instead. I usually go around 9 am on Monday and come back about 4 pm, and then go until lunch time on Tuesday unless I've got something on.*

Research suggests that older people are more likely to become involved in volunteering if asked by someone known to them, rather than through advertising (Tang & Morrow-Howell, 2008), and past involvement is a predictor of continued involvement (Morrow-Howell, 2007). This was a theme identified in all those interviewed for this chapter. Mike has volunteered with the Society of St. Vincent de Paul since age 24, when someone asked him to join. Now, at the age of 78, he still attends weekly meetings and visits the sick through this organization. Likewise, Barbara, June, and Ray have all been involved in volunteering activities within the local community for many years, although the roles that they have taken have changed over time:

> **Ray:** *I've been involved in the Scouts since I was a teenager—65 years. I've got a medal of merit for long service. I spend more time there since I retired.*
>
> **June:** *We both used to help with the camping trips and the shows. All the parents would make the costumes.*
>
> **Barbara:** *I used to help out at the church with fundraising and I was on the church cleaning rota when I was younger. I wouldn't be there [at the church shop] now if June hadn't asked me.*
>
> **June:** *Well yes, I thought you would like it and you know the people there.*

This raises the issue of attracting volunteers. If people are encouraged to consider volunteering throughout their lives as a positive use of time, it is more likely to be sustained as they enter old age. Strategies to capitalize on "word of mouth" or local community publicity should be considered as well, particularly given that research suggests that this is how many volunteers are recruited.

The continued professionalization of volunteering can deter people from continuing to volunteer in organizations due to legal requirements regarding health, safety, and training issues. This may cause withdrawal and or lessen motivation for those who have been involved in local organizations for many years. An example of this was raised by Ray:

> ...*we had a lawyer who was a member of the group and he was dead set against the national association getting their hands on [the hut that had been built by Ray and other volunteers], so he tied up the deeds so that if anything happens to this local group, it goes to the local district group. But in the last year, all the local groups have become one big group. There aren't enough commissioners who will volunteer for the job. This year, we had a £2000 (approximately $3,300) electric bill, and the insurance was £1600 (approximately $2,664). We also have to pay insurance to the London headquarters, but we don't get anything back from them. If it wasn't for the money we get from blood donor sessions we host here, it would be difficult for us to manage.*

Another area to be considered is supporting volunteers with transportation to and from the activity. In a study by Martinez, Crooks, Kim, and Tanner (2011), participants highlighted several problems with using public transportation, such as accessibility, locations that were not on bus routes, and safety if the volunteer activity occurred in the evening.

CONCLUSION

There is a plethora of writing about older people and volunteering, and this chapter has touched on only a few areas. The stories told by those interviewed mirror findings from research, highlighting the benefits gained by the volunteering activities, while acknowledging the challenges and stresses. The WHO (2007) identifies eight characteristics of "age-friendly" communities, including civic participation and employment, social participation and respect, and social inclusion, all of which relate to volunteering. Developing age-friendly communities can provide opportunities for older people to continue to participate and remain productive members of society. The older population is a rich resource that is not always recognized for the skills, knowledge, and experience they can contribute to society. They play a key role in a sustainable society, which is increasingly being recognized by policy makers. However, ways of maintaining their involvement need to be addressed. This means more than offering altruistic motivations. Volunteers want the opportunities for personal development that organized and structured volunteering can offer (Finkelstein, 2008). Consideration needs to be given, not just to what they can offer, but how they can be supported to ensure the experience of volunteering can contribute to maintaining health, quality of life, and well-being.

REFERENCES

Anheier, H. K., & Salamon, L. M., (1999). Volunteering in cross-national perspective: Initial comparisons. *Law and Contemporary Problems, 62*(4), 43-65.

Cook, J. (2011). The socio-economic contribution of older people in the UK. *Working With Older People, 15*(4), 141-146.

Davis Smith, J., & Gay, P. (2005). *Active ageing in active communities: Volunteering and the transition to retirement.* Bristol: Policy Press for the Joseph Rowntree Foundation.

Finkelstein, M. A. (2008). Predictors of volunteer time: The changing role contributions of motive fulfilment and role identity. *Social Behaviour and Personality, 36*(10), 1353-1364.

Ford, J. (2008). *Barriers to and incentives for volunteering in older people*: Research for WRVS and Ellerman Foundation, March.

Gill, Z. (2006). Older people and volunteering. *Office for Volunteers, Government of South Australia.* Retrieved December 6, 2012, from http://www.ofv.sa.gov.au/__data/assets/pdf_file/0003/8067/older-people-and-volunteering.pdf.

Lie, M., Baines, S., & Wheelock, J. (2009). Citizenship, volunteering and active ageing. *Social Policy & Administration, 43*(7), 702-718.

Longhorn, D. (2012, May 05). Donations soar after bee lady's Olympic torch moment. *Hull Daily Mail*, retrieved December 7, 2012, from http://www.thisishullandeastriding.co.uk/Donations-soar-bee-lady-s-Olympic-Torch-moment/story-16460509-detail/story.html.

Lum, T., & Lightfoot, E. (2005). The effects of volunteering on physical and mental health of older people. *Research on Aging, 27*(1), 31-55.

Martinez, I. L., Crooks, D., Kim, K. S., & Tanner, E. (2011). Invisible civic engagement among older adults: Valuing the contribution of informal volunteering. *Journal of Cross Cultural Gerontology, 26*(1), 23-37.

Morrow-Howell, N. (2007). A longer worklife: The new road to volunteering. *Aging Workforce, 31*(1), 63-67.

Morrow-Howell, N., Carden, M., & Sherraden, M., (2005). Productive engagement of older adults: Volunteerism and service. In L. Kaye (Ed.), *Perspectives on productive ageing: Social work with the new aged*. Washington, DC: NASW Press.

Morrow-Howell, N,. Hong, S., & Tang, F. (2009). Who benefits from volunteering? Variations in perceived benefits. *The Gerontologist, 49*(1), 91-102.

Parkinson, L., Warburton, J., Sibbritt, D., & Byles, J. (2010). Volunteering and older women: Psychosocial and health predictors of participation. *Aging & Mental Health, 14*(8), 917-927.

Penner, L. A., Dovidio, J. F., Piliavin, J. A., & Schroeder, D. A. (2005). Prosocial behavior: Multilevel perspectives. *Annual Review of Psychology, 56*, 365-392.

Pepin, G., & Deutscher, B. (2011). The lived experience of Australian retirees: 'I'm retired, what do I do now?' *British Journal of Occupational Therapy, 74*(9), 419-426.

Preedy, H. (2012). Volunteers: How can they work in your organization? *OT News*, 34-35.

Putnam, R. (2000). *Bowling alone: The collapse and revival of American community*. New York, NY: Simon and Schuster.

Rochester, C., & Hutchison, R. with Harris, M. & Keely, L. (2002). *A review of the Home Office Older Volunteers Initiative*. Home Office Research Study, 248. London, Home Office Research, Development and Statistics Directorate.

Tang, F. (2010). Volunteering by older adults in the United States. *China Journal of Social Work, 3*(2-3), 289-300.

Tang, F., & Morrow-Howell, N. (2008). Involvement in voluntary organizations: How older adults access volunteer roles. *Journal of Gerontological Social Work, 51*, 210-227.

Tang, F., Morrow-Howell, N., & Hong, S. (2007). *Inclusion of diverse older populations in volunteering: The role of institutional facilitation*. Presentation at the Gerontological Society of America annual meeting, San Francisco, CA.

Uglow, J. (2012, November 17). Childcare: the grandparents' army. *The Guardian*. Retrieved June 25, 2014, from http://www.theguardian.com/lifeandstyle/2012/nov/16/childcare-grandparents-army.

United States Department of Labor. (2011). Retrieved December 6, 2012, from http://www.bls.gov/news.release/volun.to1.htm.

United Kingdom Voluntary Forum. (2012). *Investing in volunteers*. Retrieved December 7, 2012, from http://iiv.investinginvolunteers.org.uk/.

University of Brighton, Age UK Brighton & Hove. (2012) Well-being in old age: findings from participatory research. Retrieved December 6, 2012, from http://eprints.brighton.ac.uk/10631/1/Well_being_in_old_age_findings_from_participatory_research_full_report.pdf.

Van Dyne, L., & Farmer, S. M. (2005). It's who I am: Role identity and organizational citizenship behaviour of volunteers. In D. L. Turnipseed (Ed.), *Handbook of organizational citizenship behavior: A review of 'good soldier' activity in organizations* (pp. 177-203). New York: Nova Science Publishers.

Warburton, J. (2006). Volunteering in later life: Is it good for your health? *Voluntary Action, 8*, 3-15.

Warburton, J., & Jeppsson Grassman, E. (2009). Variations in older people's social and productive ageing activities across different social welfare regimes. *International Journal of Social Welfare, 20*(2), 180-191.

Warburton, J., Paynter, J., & Petriwskyj, A. (2007). Volunteering as a productive aging activity: Incentives and barriers to volunteering by Australian seniors. *Journal of Applied Gerontology, 26*(4), 333-354.

Watts, A. (1977). *The essence of Alan Watts*. Millbrae: Celestial Arts.

Wilson, J. (2000). Volunteering. *Annual Review of Sociology, 26*, 215-240.

World Health Organization. (2007). *Global age-friendly cities: A guide*. Retrieved December 13, 2012, from http://www.who.int/ageing/publications/Global_age_friendly_cities_Guide_English.pdf.

WRVS. (2011) *Gold age pensioners: Valuing the socio-economic contribution of older people in the UK*. Retrieved September 4, 2013, from http://www.royalvoluntaryservice.org.uk/Uploads/Documents/gold_age_report_2011.pdf.

Technology's Impact on the Way Older People Work and Socialize

Laura Dimmler, PhD, MHA; Erin E. Hunt, BS; and Caroline Wolverson, DipCOT, DipHT, MSc

Try to become not a man of success, but try rather to become a man of value.—Albert Einstein (Miller, 1955)

INTRODUCTION

This chapter will consider the use of technology in its widest form. Not only the use of information and communication technologies, which include computer-based devices and the internet, but also assistive technology (AT). AT can be defined as "an umbrella term for any device or system that allows individuals to perform tasks they would otherwise be unable to do or increases the ease and safety with which tasks can be performed" (World Health Organization, 2004). A further definition from the Kings Fund Centre (2001) focuses on the role of AT in maximizing independence: "any product or service designed to enable independence for disabled and older people."

Although research regarding the adaptability and use of technology by older people is not new, our understanding of their adoption and use of technology is still limited (Computer Supported Cooperative Work Conference, 2011). It is recognized that digital technologies can have a positive impact on the process of aging and the way older people work, however, among the various populations of technology users, demographic variables can influence adaptability and use. These variables include age, income, education, and race, with those who are younger, wealthier, more educated, and White demonstrating greater access to and use of technology for both work and entertainment (Lorence, Park, & Fox, 2006; Porter & Donthu, 2006; Zickuhr & Smith, 2012).

Steggell, Hooker, Bowman, Brandt, and Lee (2007) found that culture and personal experience also influence technology acceptance by individuals. The attitudes and values of individual users, such as independence and the perceived unreliability of certain technologies, have an impact on the adoption of technology and may impact on the individual's ability to maintain their work role

Hunt LA, Wolverson C.
Work and the Older Person: Increasing Longevity and Well-Being (pp 113-123).
© 2015 SLACK Incorporated.

effectively. Despite this, the accessibility of technology for older people, while offering challenges, can give rise to many opportunities to maintain independence and employment.

This chapter covers interviews with older people describing how they have been introduced to technology throughout their lives and the importance it now holds for them in maintaining a productive lifestyle. The first narrative from 27-year-old Erin Hunt, who works at a agency specializing in web design, web development, e-commerce, mobile app development, and digital marketing. She reflects on her work as a creative director/user experience lead and considers her experiences of growing up with technology and designing technology for others' use:

> *In my career as a creative director and user experience lead, I am constantly working with new technologies. As the web grows, so does the vast amount of programs and applications. At times, I find it exhilarating and wonderfully rewarding to learn about all the latest new technologies, but at the same time, in a world where technology changes vastly on a quarterly basis, it can be frightening and overwhelming.*
>
> *For me, there is less of a learning curve. My whole life I've been learning how to operate new technologies and write new programming languages. I've grown up with this constant need to stay current in a world that is constantly changing, and fortunately, I've had success with this. I've been trained and conditioned to expect this change. But for many older people, these rapid technology updates can cause major issues in the work force. "In a report published by the Society of Human Resource Management (SHRM), the largest obstacle cited to hiring older workers is that they do not keep up with current technology"* (Spiezle, 2005).
>
> *This disconnect between older people and technology can occur for both psychological and physical reasons. For example, certain psychological variables, such as anxiety about technology or self-efficiency, are better predictors than age or previous experience* (Jung et al., 2010).
>
> *In addition, as we age, our motor skills may be affected by coordination problems, weakness, or reaction time. For some older people, the presence of a motor difficulty had a negative effect on their ability to perform well on certain computer tasks* (Fezzani, Albinet, Thon, & Marquié, 2010). *"As our population lives and works longer, the likelihood of developing age-related vision, hearing, and dexterity impairments increase as we approach 40. These changes directly affect the aging workers' ability to use computing devices. For some they may be an inconvenience, while for others they may become disabling"* (Spiezle, 2005).
>
> *Luckily, there are modifications people in my field can do to make user interfaces more welcoming to older people. And easy enough, these tweaks that are beneficial for the older person are also beneficial for the population at large. Many of these issues can be addressed by size. Using a large font size, and creating contrast between foreground text and the background is key to good legibility. Hwang, Williams, and Batson (2008) found that by using targets that expand to a larger size, giving user a larger area to click on, elders were able to "point and click" faster and make fewer mistakes.*
>
> *For interfaces that are specifically for older people, using animations to ensure that the user knows the effect of every action can be helpful. Mitchell in* UX Magazine *explains boomers grew up in an analog world, where mechanical actions begat mechanical responses....Think of how when you download an app on iOS, you're taken to the homescreen and forced to watch the app download. True, this often frustrates power users, but for a child of the analog age, it links cause and effect in a clear and understandable manner. (http://uxmag.com/articles/romancing-the-boomer).*
>
> *As the baby boomers age and continue working into their later years, both they, their employers, and those using creative interfaces need to adapt. For the aging population, staying current with technology is crucial. Technology has become so intertwined into the world. This population needs to embrace these new tools both in their professional and personal lives. I tell older people to go ahead—get the latest and greatest iPhone.*

For employers, ongoing technology training should be mandatory for all employees. For interface designers, we need to keep older people in mind when designing. Creating something new is always fun, but it isn't always the most beneficial to our users especially those that like routines and sticking to habits learned over the years.

CHALLENGES TO ADOPTION OF TECHNOLOGY

Increasingly, technology is being used by older people to enable them to remain independent, but the complexity of technology design often stifles older people (Nielsen-Norman Group, 2013). In their recent study, 45% of older people indicated that they were hesitant to explore and uncomfortable trying new things. When using technology, older people also were more than twice as likely to give up on a task if they failed to achieve it the first time. To build confidence and encourage technology use, technology manufacturers should offer supportive designs, avoid design changes, and provide easily readable instructions. As an example, wireless technology is well accepted by older people because it is seamless and supports independent living. Employers should also consider how technology is introduced within the workplace, keeping these considerations in mind for older workers.

Erin's experience (previous) highlights the importance of involving older people in the design of technology systems. Sheldon (2014, p. 176) argues for effective regulation to ensure organizations focus on accessible technology. She states that barriers to access are often created through discriminatory design as disabled people are not 'designed in' to products and as a consequence need to purchase expensive additional equipment. This is echoed by Pedlow, Kasnitz and Shuttleworth (2010) in their study of cell phone use by older people with impairments. They found that although appropriate technology exists, it is not put together effectively to support this client group, even by companies that focus on older people with disabilities. One way to address this is having older people on design teams—providing them with employment opportunities and also ensuring that technology meets their needs.

Using the technology acceptance model (TAM) in their research design, Porter and Donthu (2006) found that despite the fact that most Americans use the Internet, factors such as age, education, income, and race were associated differentially with beliefs about it and that these beliefs influence a consumer's attitude toward and use of the Internet. In addition, this research also indicated that although access barriers can be significant, perceptions about the ease of use and personal relevance of the technology to an individual's life have a stronger effect than demographics alone.

An increasing number of older people in the workforce where younger managers may have five generations working together is leading to a paradigm shift in the way young people lead in an intergenerational setting (Haeger & Lingham, 2013). Their study found that while older workers were expecting a people-centered approach by managers to leadership, younger people in leadership roles were adopting task-centered or results-centered approaches. Naturally, where this incongruence occurs, there are strained interactions plus, it would be expected, a reduction in productivity.

In their study, Haeger and Lingham (2013) identified the pace and use of technology as areas of conflict. They found that older workers resisted juggling so many tasks in a day while admiring what leaders were able to achieve. In addition, the study identified frustration by older workers, for example:

> *"We can't even do a simple ID card anymore because they're all bar-coded."*
> *"If I have a question about something that's electronic, I wait till I get home and I might call a friend to try to figure out what I'm trying to figure out because less and less—I feel less and less comfortable in the office."* (p. 294)

This can result in loss of self-esteem, confidence in the workplace, and damage to well-being while leading to frustration on the part of leaders as identified by one:

> *"He still does his billing on a scrap piece of paper and just writes it all down, a sticker of the patient identification, and hands it to the senior AA to fill out the billing. The other guys are more self-sufficient. They're younger." (p. 294)*

This blanket assumption that it is age impacting ability to embrace new technology, may lead to social distance (dictionary.com)—the distance that is placed between ourselves and those we see as different from us, which can lead to the growth of prejudice and ultimately discrimination within the workplace.

The *digital divide*—socioeconomic and other disparities that keep individuals from benefiting from technological resources—is another barrier to access and according to Neves (2012), there is still a significant age-based digital divide. In a follow-up study to Pew's 2000 Internet and American Life Project, Zickuhr and Smith (2012) found that significant differences in use remain, which generally are related to age, household income, and educational attainment.

Another interesting perspective regarding the use of technology by older people is the parallel link of these variables to the social determinants of health. The social determinants of health—the economic and social conditions in which individuals live—determine the wellness or illness of each individual, and are similar to those variables that influence technology adaptation and use. These social determinant variables include age, socioeconomic status, education, social structures, and economic systems (Centers for Disease Control and Prevention, 2013). Because technology is becoming more integral to health-related activities and access to health information across populations, the parallel between technology adoption and social determinant variables is intriguing (Kreps & Beckjord, 2009).

Barriers to utilizing information technology can have an impact on health, and as a consequence people's ability to work. Different institutional structures influence the development and diffusion of technology and with the added impetus of health care reform in the U.S., technological developments related to the care of older people are causing a shift in decision making and resource allocation away from physicians and administrators to patients and families. These developments are placing pressure on institutional structures and individuals, and shaping the development of new technologies. These various pressures, innovations, and the divergent uptake of new technologies are significant for older people because these ultimately determine institutional advantage for technology development and diffusion, impacting on quality, cost, and access to health care, and the ability of individuals to remain healthy and independent as they age (Gingrich, 2012), and through this, maintain a productive lifestyle.

According to Gingrich (2012), use of technology among older people and rates of diffusion of consumer-oriented medical technology has been slow in the United States. These differential rates of technology uptake are influenced by social structures and determine diffusion of new technology to end-users, such as ATs to older people. Social structures that maintain centralized administration of technology reduce access. In the U.S., this means that older people may be required to pay more for ATs and not have access to leading-edge technology (Gingrich, 2012).

Sheldon (2014) argues that everyday information and communication technology that is now in the working environment is changing the way we live and alongside this, the social category of the people we consider 'disabled'. While the use of technology can offer opportunities for enablement, at the same time can be disabling for those who find it difficult to adapt to its use in ever increasing technology-dependent work environments. Sheldon (2014, p. 175) further highlights the importance of not using technology as a 'sticking plaster' solution to deeper social problems.

EMBRACING TECHNOLOGICAL ADVANCES

It should be recognized, that despite these challenges, many older people embrace the use of technologies to enhance their home and work environments. Recent statistical reports demonstrate that older adults are the fastest growing segment among internet users (Organization for Economic Co-operation and Development, 2011; Pew Internet and American Life Project, 2010). Studies demonstrate that learning computer and internet skills enhance a sense of independence (Henke, 1999) and create a process of empowerment as a result of the power of change and the power of knowledge (Shapira, Barak, & Gal, 2007). In addition, internet use is associated with strengthened self-image and self-confidence, higher levels of social connectivity, higher levels of perceived social support, decreased feelings of loneliness, lower levels of depression, and generally more positive attitudes toward aging (Dickenson & Hill, 2007; Fokkema & Knipscheer, 2007; Van de Watering, 2005). Nimrod (2013) suggests that internet use may play a significant role in successful aging.

Fiona's story, demonstrates how the lifelong use of technology continues to contribute to quality of life and wellbeing:

> Fiona has lived in the same area her entire life. She graduated from high school in 1958, taking many college-prep, decision making, and quantitative courses, before continuing her education at a state university. She is a self-described lifelong learner. After leaving college, Fiona's first job was working as a secretary for a bank; the things she liked best about her job were the opportunities for continuing education, advancing her career, and learning new technologies.
>
> Her initial job with the bank involved little technology; she was responsible for preparing correspondence, using only shorthand and a typewriter. However, in 1958, her employer began offering VISA cards to consumers, Fiona's new career was launched when her supervisor offered her a position issuing credit cards to customers. She quickly advanced from a clerk to a supervisor, witnessing the rapid expansion of technology across the banking sector and the transformation it brought.
>
> With the introduction of ATMs in 1969, her employer found that customers were reluctant to use them. Fiona's supervisor guessed that this might be caused by a breakdown in communication between the technicians who developed the ATMs and the people at the bank who understood what consumers wanted. Again, he called on Fiona because he needed someone who understood the needs of the bank's customers.
>
> By the mid-1970s, Fiona's career was definitively linked to technology when she was transferred to automate loan payment processing. "I didn't have any formal training in programming or computer technology, but I was selected for this assignment over all the male programming staff because of my experience in customer service, and my supervisor felt I was a quick study. He knew I understood the importance of the human interface with technology," said Fiona. In this new job, she tested computer equipment and worked with the programmers to make adjustments more suited to consumer needs. Fiona said, "To do my job effectively, I had to learn how everything worked and the way that programmers think. In the process, I became absolutely fearless of technology." As the machines were tested and distributed across U.S. Bank's system, customers and staff needed training, and this became another new job for Fiona.
>
> Fiona was the bank's lead trainer for the next six years, traveling three to four times a year to deliver more training as computer technology saturated the banking industry. In addition to training bank tellers, customer service staff, and executive managers, Fiona was tasked with training the bank's programmers as well, traveling more to bank branches out of state as services expanded. She taught staff how to use new phone systems as well as computers. "I developed all of this training from whole cloth. Nothing had been developed

before I took over the role as trainer," said Fiona. When she was back at the office, Fiona spent most of her time taking calls from staff and programmers, improvising solutions to technical problems they presented to her. She would then apply this new expertise to update and improve the training programs she developed. As technology continued to evolve, Fiona continued working as a technology trainer for her employer, and in 1989 she was put in charge of training all staff for the bank's 24-hour call center system. In the late 1980s, the staff training Fiona had developed was replicated because with the training in place, call centers experienced a very low turnover rate of less than five percent. It was during this period at the call center that Fiona interacted with a personal computer for the first time. "I taught myself how to use the PC to prepare spreadsheets, and I also learned other PC applications," she said. Fiona's life experiences taught her to be "absolutely fearless of technology."

Fiona retired in 1994, after spending 25 years with her employer. So how does Fiona's life-time experience adapting and using technology influence her perspective on technology in her day-to-day activities, now that she is retired? When she was asked this question, Fiona felt that her parents instilled in her a "can-do" attitude about life, so she always felt she could get anything done. Throughout her life, Fiona believed she could be successful with anything she put her mind to, and this included using technology. She could always figure it out, so learning about and using new technology never intimidated her. Fiona also believes that her successes with technology gave her an enthusiasm to try new things. Today, Fiona has a PC and a smart phone, blogs regularly with a friend from high school, and prepares desktop publications for her church. She taught herself how to use the publishing software.

Fiona's lifelong interest in technology has enabled her to continue to use this tool to maintain a productive lifestyle contributing to her quality of life and well-being into retirement. Fiona's story also highlights the importance of the human interface with technology.

Porter and Donthu (2006) use the TAM to help explain why differences in technology use may exist. This is important because the TAM identifies prevalent attitudes regarding ease of use and usefulness as primary determinants of an individual's use of technology, regardless of population demographics; this finding has been confirmed by the Pew Internet Report (2010), Morris (2005), Suchman (1994), and the Nielsen-Norman Group (2013). All of those interviewed for this chapter, believe that technology is very useful in their personal and work lives and that it is easy to use. However, they began using technology early in their careers at a time when it was becoming an integral tool for business, entertainment, and personal use. More research is needed to determine how external variables such as access barriers, might also influence the adoption of technology use by specific populations, including older people, particularly those who do not have the advantage of income and education to ease transition to technology use as aging occurs.

Within the work environment, Skirbekk (2003) found that there is prejudice against older people in the workplace, which causes discrimination. However, the research also indicates that older people are not incompetent or technophobes when it comes to using technology. Employers rate older workers better in attendance, punctuality, productivity, and performance, particularly when tasks require greater experience, verbal abilities, and interest in learning to use technology with proficiency.

Technology can play a dualistic role in the work and social lives of older people (Suchman, 1994). It may increase social isolation, but technology also has the capacity to alleviate it. Social disengagement can increase with the physical and cognitive decline of aging, but new technologies can enhance awareness and control of social engagement, fostering empowerment and social health (Morris, 2005). Social activity, especially among older people, is a significant indicator and predictor of health status. New technologies can create social networks and support an individual's sense of self, independent functioning in daily activities, and physical health (Morris, 2005). Being introduced to technology in the work place is likely to enhance and encourage the use of technology outside of the workplace. This is demonstrated by the stories of Hannah and Michelle:

Hannah graduated from nursing school and became a nursing cadet in 1950. After serving 22 months with the military, she was hired by a hospital where she was assigned the responsibility of setting up the first surgical recovery room in the state. After more than ten years at this hospital, Hannah moved to take a nursing supervisor position. She arrived there during the implementation of the hospital's first electronic health record system. As a result, her first steps included extensive computer training. "In nursing school, I was trained as a bedside nurse, spending time with patients and doctors; but because of technology, nursing does not look the same today," said Hannah. "Now nurses do mostly paperwork and supervise other staff, so you lose the relationships with patients and families. You know the patient's background as a result of the technology—the symptoms, the problems, and the demographics—but no relationships. Before when there was a death, we were right there with the family."

Today Hannah has a cell phone, uses books on tape, and has a computer for e-mail and music. "My grand-daughter lives in Australia, and e-mail is how I keep in touch with her," she said. "I think technology is really important, but not enough people have gone deeper into technology to understand the impact on people and relationships," said Hannah. "I think technology is great, but not for people my age because relationships are so much more important."

Hannah's story highlights the need to consider the impact of technology on relationships and that although it is no replacement for social contacts; it has the potential to enhance these.

Michelle was born in a small farming community; she graduated from high school in 1959 and was married that July. Despite her roots in a remote rural community, Michelle traveled the world when her husband joined the Marine Corps. When they returned to the United States in 1963, her husband was offered a job as a police officer.

Michelle's first job when returning home was working as a waitress, but soon she was offered a new position as a sales clerk at a department store. After several years with this company, Michelle took a job as a sales representative for another department store, and spent more than 20 years with them

After many years as a police officer, Michelle's husband decided to attend law school and this was the impetus for Michelle to learn how to use a computer; her husband needed someone to type his homework for him, so in the evenings this was Michelle's second job. At the same time, computers were being introduced into the workplace so as her career advanced from sales to the inventory and pricing department, it became a necessity for Michelle to develop her computer skills. Working in the inventory and pricing department for more than five years, it was her responsibility to conduct computer audits, checking various accounts for accuracy. Michelle taught herself how to use the accounting software on weekends when she was not regularly scheduled to work. "When I was working inventory, my supervisor would tell me that it was the best inventory audit they ever had. I had to learn a lot, but by the end of my five years there, I knew a lot," she said. So they assigned her to oversee inventory in four departments including small electronics, sporting goods, lawn and garden, and hardware and home improvement. "I had to learn the technology in each department, from TVs and telephones to installing ceiling fans and water heaters, so I could inventory all the parts," said Michelle. As part of a cross-training requirement, Michelle also learned how to use the company switchboard.

Michelle retired in 1996, but she already had bought her first home computer in 1992 without a modem, then she bought a second one with a modem in 1993 so she could track her family's ancestry online. "I am not against the evolution of technology," said Michelle. "It's made our lives easier and it makes my brain work." Today Michelle has a cell phone, a PC with a wireless printer, an iPad with a keyboard that is connected to the Internet via WiFi, and she manages all of her finances online. Michelle uses the iPad to play games and record her family's ancestry which she has tracked back to the early 1700s. "Throughout my life, I have never been intimidated by technology," she said. "You don't think about it, you just do it."

Michelle exemplifies someone who, although now retired, maintains a productive lifestyle through the use of technology. It is evident that the three individuals interviewed for this chapter are not average technology users, given their age, education, and socioeconomic status. However, these narratives support the findings that education, income, and race influence the adoption and use of technology. All of the older people interviewed for this chapter are White, college educated, and have a middle-class or upper middle-class socioeconomic rank.

Van de Watering (2013) identifies how technology can increase cognitive ability and decrease feelings of loneliness in older people as they age through the use of computer games and e-mail and this is again highlighted in the stories told here. Yet, as has been discussed earlier in this chapter, to achieve this, a number of access barriers need to be addressed, including modifications to make technology less cumbersome to use, removing anxiety toward technology, and demonstrating that it is relevant to older people. This can be accomplished with design changes that include universal design and accessibility, and improving computer-based communication in a way that can positively impact older people and society at large. The positive outcomes that might be achieved with such changes include greater personal independence, the ability to communicate, retrieve information and remain socially engaged, and an increased feeling of satisfaction with life (Kaye, 2011) and also the opportunity to remain in the workplace for longer. Technology also may enable older people to remain working via home computer systems, providing more opportunities to work from home or be self-employed, however, although this may meet financial needs, the challenge of remaining socially connected when working from home must be considered. There is also a need to better understand the limitations experienced by special user groups, such as individuals with disabilities, when adopting technology.

ATs offer a means of older people remaining in the workplace. This has been discussed in Chapters 5 and 7. It is important for employers and employees to work together to ensure that technology is appropriate to meet their needs and that the individual is appropriately assessed to ensure time and money are not wasted.

For those with more specialist, individual needs a UK charity, REMAP (http://www.remap.org.uk/) provides individual items of AT supporting people to maintain their independence in aspects of self-care, leisure, and productivity. An example of this is the case of Anne, who following an accident, was left with weakness in her wrist affecting her ability to manipulate the screw tops on test tubes in her job in microbiology. Remap designed a device to hold the test tubes, leaving her able to unscrew them with her unaffected hand. There are other similar organizations throughout the world such as TAD in Australia (http://www.tadaustralia.org.au/) and TETRA Society in North America (http://www.tetrasociety.org/). TETRA have made a minor adaptation for Shara Gutscher in the workplace. Following a brain injury she was left with limited vision and only able to use her right arm. Shara works for a company renting out 2 way radios to film companies. Gregg Harris who works for TETRA created a wooden cradle and clamp to hold the radios enabling Shara to check and clean the radios (http://www.tetrasociety.org/about/testimonies.php). Although not an older person, this is an example of how a minor piece of AT could enable someone to remain productive.

Many of those volunteering for such organizations are retired themselves, often from a health profession background, or like Ken Kirwood of TAD who is a retired joiner and carpenter who has been involved in the organization in New South Wales for 13 years, ensuring he maintains a productive lifestyle and continues to contribute to his community and society.

Suchman's (1994) research supports the need to resolve technology barriers, and defines it as "self-evident technology" that can be grasped at first sight. Suchman indicates that the adoption and use of technology requires a socialization process where it is incorporated into the performance of daily activities. This process is expedited if the individual possesses greater technological acumen and is supported by various social structures including family, the media, and other institutions such as the work environment.

User experience (UX) is how a person feels when interacting with a website, mobile application, or any human-computer system. Does this website give value? Can viewers find what they are seeking? Is it pleasant to use? There are many things a UX designer can design to ensure that their users are successful. In particular, when designing interfaces for older adults, there are two key items to keep in mind (Fezzani, Albinet, Thon, & Marquié, 2010):

1. Visual acuity: Beginning in the early to mid-forties, most adults may start to experience problems with their ability to see clearly at close distances, especially for reading and computer tasks.

2. Motor skills: As people age, their motor skills may be affected by coordination problems, weakness, or reaction time. For some older people, the presence of motor difficulty may result in poor ability to perform certain computer tasks.

These physical changes can directly affect the aging workers' ability to use computing devices (Spiezle, 2005). For some individuals, this may be an inconvenience, but for others these losses could become disabling (Spiezle, 2005). Impairments with computer interfacing may even result in work abandonment.

Fortunately, there are an increasing number of modifications to support older people, for example, interfaces that are specifically for older people, using animations to ensure that the user knows the effect of every action can be helpful. Mitchell in *UX Magazine* (2013) explains boomers grew up in an analog world, where mechanical actions begat mechanical responses. UX designers can use this to their advantage when designing for older adults by ensuring that they use a similar cause and effect approach (http://uxmag.com/articles/romancing-the-boomer).

For the aging population, staying current with technology is crucial. Technology has become so intertwined into the world and it is easy to get behind. This population needs to embrace these new tools both in their professional and personal lives. By breaking habits with new updated programs, they learn new information that may stimulate cognition. For interface designers, they need to keep older people in mind when designing. Creating something new is always fun, but it is not always the most beneficial to users, especially those that like routines and sticking to habits learned over the years. Changes need to make logical sense to older technology consumers and involving older people in the design process is one way to address this.

Conclusion

Research regarding the effects of income and age relating to online information seeking has been inconsistent. In a recent study conducted by Nielsen (2013), the primary uses of technology by older people included seeking and managing health information, finances, and social activities. Eastman and Iyer (2004) demonstrate that older consumers have favorable intentions toward using computers and the internet; most learn to use the internet on their own, and they would prefer to learn more about the internet if they had access to classes at convenient locations. With the increasing numbers of older people remaining in work, it is likely that this balance will change and introduction to technology and use of the internet, will often be taking place within the work environment encouraging people to transfer skills to the home environment—as in the case of the three people who have told their stories in this chapter. Evidence shows that those older people with higher levels of income are more willing to both use the internet and purchase products online.

There is perhaps a tendency by society to think of technology and the use of computers as a recent event but those who have told their stories in this chapter demonstrate that it is this older generation who have played a key role in the introduction of technology within the workplace.

Nevertheless, a number of issues have been raised in this chapter with regard to both opportunities and barriers for older people using technology within their homes and work lives. The interface with new technology may not be intuitive to many of the current older generation. New technology is often created by a younger generation who may have a different approach. The importance of intergenerational working and consideration of universal design is imperative, as highlighted by Erin Hunt who told her story at the start of this chapter. Training and time provided to learn how to use new technology is the key for successful usage by all, not just older people in the workplace.

Society as a whole, and more specifically employers, need to consider how worker success with technology can be achieved, particularly with the current generation of older people, many of whom are unfamiliar with some of the newer technologies. ATs have the potential to prolong the working lives of older people by increasing flexibility; for example, where a job can be done and also by reducing physical effort such as the opportunity for paperless offices. These opportunities should be embraced to become the norm for all workers, not just older people; however, the consequence will be to provide enhanced opportunity for maintenance of a productive lifestyle into old age.

REFERENCES

Computer Supported Cooperative Work Conference. (2011). Socialising technology among older people in Asia. March 19-23, 2011. Hangzhou, China.

Dickenson A., & Hill R. L. (2007). Keeping in touch: Talking to older people about computers and communication. *Educational Gerontology, 33,* 613-630.

Dictonary.com. (2014). Retrieved March 3, 2014, from http://dictionary.reference.com/browse/social+distance.

Eastman, J., & Iyer, R. (2004). Older people's uses and attitudes towards the Internet. *Journal of Consumer Marketing, 21*(3), 208-220.

Fezzani, K., Albinet, C., Thon, B., & Marquie, J. C. (2010). The effect of motor difficulty on the acquisition of a computer task: a comparison between young and older adults. *Behaviour and Information Technology, 29*(2), 115-124.

Fokkema, T., & Knipscheer K. (2007). Escape loneliness by going digital: A quantitative and qualitative evaluation of a Dutch experiment in using ECT to overcome loneliness among older adults. *Aging & Mental Health, 11,* 496–504.

Gingrich, J. (2012). Health and elderly care technology. The Berkeley Roundtable on the International Economy (BRIE), University of California at Berkeley. Retrieved January 18, 2013, from http://brie.berkeley.edu/publications/Health%20and%20elderly%20care%20technology.pdf.

Haeger, D. L., & Lingham, T. (2013). Intergenerational collisions and leadership in the 21st century. *Journal of Intergenerational Relationships, 11,* 286-303. Retrieved March 4, 2014, from http://www.tandfonline.com/doi/abs/10.1080/15350770.2013.810525#.Uxb1OFRFDcs.

Henke, M. (1999). Promoting independence in older persons through the Internet. *CyberPsychology & Behavior, 2,* 521-527.

Hwang, F., Williams, N., & Batson, H. (2008). Improving computer interaction for older users: Investigating dynamic on-screen targets. Retrieved September 18, 2013, from www.sparc.ac.uk/media/downloads/.../exec_summary_hwang.pdf.

Jung, Y., Peng, W., Meghan, M., Jin, S., Jordan-Marsh, M., McLaughlin, M.L., & Silverstein, M. (2010). Low-income minority seniors' enrollment in a cyber cafe: Psychological barriers to crossing the digital divide. *Educational Gerontology. 36*(3), 193-212.

Kaye, J. (2011). Putting petabytes to work: Home-based assessment technology can help elders manage their health. *Aging Today, 32*(1), 1-2.

Kings Fund Centre. (2001). Consultation Meeting on Assistive Technology. London: Kings Fund.

Kreps, G., and Beckjord, E. (2009). Using the Internet for health-related activities: Findings from a national probability sample. *Journal of Medical Internet Research, 11*(1). Retrieved February 11, 2013, from http://www.ncbi.nlm.nih.gov/pmc/articles/PMC2762768/#ref10.

Lorence, D., Park, H., & Fox S. (2006). Assessing health consumerism on the Web: A demographic profile of information-seeking behaviors. *Journal of Medical Systems, 4,* 251-258.

Miller, W. (1955, May 2). Death of a genius: His fourth dimension, time, overtakes einstein. *LIFE, 38.*

Mitchell, S. (2013). Romancing the Boomer: Designing apps that resonate with older users. Retrieved September 1, 2013, from http://uxmag.com/articles/romancing-the-boomer.

Morris, M. (2005). Social networks as health feedback displays. *Internet Computing, September-October,* 29-37.

Neves, B. (2012). Too old for technology? How older people of Lisbon use and perceive information and communication technologies. *Journal of Community Informatics, 8*(1), 1712-1741.

Nielsen-Norman Group. (2013). Evidence-based User Experience Research: Usability for senior citizens. Retrieved April 13, 2013, from http://www.nngroup.com/articles/usability-for-senior-citizens/.

Nimrod, G. (2013). Probing the audience of seniors' online communities. *Journals of Gerontology: Series B, 68*(5), 773-782.

Organization for Economic Co-operation and Development (OECD). (2011). *The future of the Internet economy: A statistical profile*. Retrieved September 10, 2013, from http://www.oecd.org/internet/ieconomy/48255770.pdf.

Pedlow, R., Kasnitz, D., & Shuttleowrth, R. (2010). Barriers to the adoption of cell phones for older people with impairments in the USA: Results from an expert review and field study. *Technology and Disability, 22*, 147-158.

Pew Internet and American Life Project (PIALP). (2010). Four in ten seniors go online. Retrieved September 10, 2013, from http://www.pewinternet.org/Commentary/2010/January/38-of-adults-age-65-go-online.aspx.

Porter, C., & Donthu, N. (2006). Using the technology acceptance model to explain how attitudes determine Internet usage: The role of perceived access barriers and demographics. *Journal of Business Research, 59*, 999-1007.

Shapira, N., Barak, A., & Gal, I. (2007). Promoting older adults' well being through Internet training and use. *Aging and Mental Health, 11*, 477-484.

Sheldon, A. (2014). Changing Technology. In J. Swain., S. French., C. Barnes & C. Thomas. *Disabling Barriers – Enabling Environments* (pp. 173-180). London: Sage Publications Ltd.

Skirbekk, V. (2003). Age and individual productivity: A literature survey. Max Planck Institute for Demographics.

Spiezle, C. (2005). Convergence of technology, aging & employability. Retrieved June 4, 2014, from http://www.age-light.com/webdocs/Convergence%20of%20Technology,%20Aging%20&%20Employability.pdf.

Steggell, C., Hooker, K., Bowman, S., Brandt, J., & Lee, M. (2007). Acceptance of gerotechnologies by older women in rural areas. Oregon State University. Presentation at the Second International Conference on Technology and Aging, Toronto, Ontario, Canada.

Suchman, L. (1994). *Plans and situated actions: The problem of human machine communication*. New York, NY: University of Cambridge Press.

Van de Watering, M. (2013). The impact of technology on older people. *The December Years*. Retrieved January 18, 2013, from http://decemberyears.org/the-impact-of-computer-technology-on- the-elderly/.

World Health Organization. (2004). *Glossary Of Terms For Community Health Care And Services For Older Persons*. Cited Foundation for Assistive Technology (FAST) retrieved January 9, 2014, from http://fastuk.org/about/definitionofat.php.

Zickuhr, K., & Smith, A. (2012). PEW Internet Report: Digital Differences. Retrieved January 23, 2013, from: http://pewinternet.org/Reports/2012/Digital-differences.aspx.

11

Finding New Work and Reinventing Oneself

Marian Arbesman, PhD, OTR/L

Nobody grows old merely by living a number of years. We grow old by deserting our ideals. Years may wrinkle the skin, but to give up enthusiasm wrinkles the soul.—Samuel Ullman (n.d.)

With advancing age, it is common to consider whether all career goals have been achieved. During this process of re-evaluation, the idea of career reinvention may be contemplated. Through the use of narratives, this chapter explores the characteristics of individuals who reinvent themselves, and why they engage in this process. In addition, the chapter includes resources to support people in this pursuit.

Typically, reinvention is thought of as remaking oneself or making oneself over in a different form. Definitions of reinvention, however, may also include the concept of bringing back or reviving earlier interests (dictionary.com, 2013).

Reinventing work with older people, also known as re-careering or encore careers (Freedman, 2008), takes many forms. Feldman (2002) distinguishes between job change—where one moves to a different position within an organization—and career change, or "entry into a new occupation which requires fundamentally different skills, daily routines, and work environments from the present one" (Feldman, 2002, p. 76). An older person may stay in the same career, but may change part of his or her work responsibilities (e.g., someone who leaves a management position to have day-to-day contact with customers). In another scenario, an older person may build on present or past skills and knowledge to go into a different area (e.g., someone working for a large retail bookstore may decide to set up an online store selling books targeted to those interested in travel). While many of the skills this individual had honed over the years would be useful for the online presence, other skills need to be developed in order to make the venture successful. An example of this is Keith Oliver, a retired head teacher diagnosed with dementia who now reviews books on dementia and has helped to set up the Alzheimer's Society reading resource. He is also involved in raising public awareness of Dementia (Alzheimer's Society, 2013). Keith's full story is available on YouTube, http://www.youtube.com/watch?v=CPulwcrkcxA.

- 125 -

Hunt LA, Wolverson C.
Work and the Older Person: Increasing Longevity and Well-Being (pp 125-134).
© 2015 SLACK Incorporated.

In another scenario, an individual may go into a totally different area from his or her previous work. This is demonstrated by Philip Zuber, who was made redundant from a senior executive post after working for the same company for 34 years:

I spent a month in full-time retirement. I was really despondent. At 52, it was hard to be told that you'd reached your use-by date. I was afraid of being rejected. I'd heard an awful lot about people of my age applying for hundreds of jobs and not getting anywhere. I felt I was about to enter a competition where the odds were against me. To be honest, I was used to sitting on the other side of the table employing people.

For the last 2 years, Philip has been working in the homes of the elderly and people with disabilities, carrying out repairs and making modifications. He says his age and experience has been an enormous advantage when it comes to working with a diverse group of clients.

I've got the ability to slow down and have time for people these days. I'm not sure I would have been able to do that in my younger years—I always had too much to do.

I used to go into the same office every day, but no 2 days are the same here. I love taking in all the new information. It's incredibly stimulating.

I have some physical limitations at my age, and some of the younger fellows don't have the skills, but that's the benefit of having a balanced team—there's no job we can't do when we put our ideas and experiences together. (Australian Human Rights Commission, 2008)

An individual who has a long-held dream and decides to fulfill that dream in later life is also in this category. Perhaps someone who worked in business for many years always dreamed of helping at-risk children. During this individual's encore career, he sets up an after-school program for children living in his neighborhood.

The U.S. Small Business Administration (SBA) and American Association of Retired Persons (AARP) are also involved in helping retirees into encore careers as entrepreneurs (http://www.sba.gov/about-sba-services/7367/554261). For example, Linda Lombri and Virginia Cornue, in their postretirement lives, have reinvented themselves as mystery writers and entrepreneurs, even though neither had written fiction before. They began an e-book series, the *Sandra Troux Mysteries,* which is sold on 10 websites, including Amazon, Barnes & Noble, and iTunes. The first in the series, *The Mystery of the Ming Connection,* was published last year under their pseudonym, Crystal Sharpe.

RESEARCH ON CAREER REINVENTION

Who Reinvents?

Research has examined the characteristics of older people who develop a new career path. Johnson, Kawachi, and Lewis (2009) used data from the Health and Retirement Survey on 51- to 55-year-old individuals working full-time in 1992 who were followed up in 2006 at ages 65 to 69. By 2006, 80% had changed jobs, and half of all workers who left their jobs had a new employer. Two-thirds of those switching jobs (and 27% of all older workers) had changed occupations. Further analysis indicated that older workers and those who did not complete high school were significantly less likely to change careers than those individuals who graduated from high school and did not attend any college. Individuals with defined benefit pension coverage were less likely to leave a job.

The impact of present work on other life activities also determines retirement age and interest in moving towards a new job or career. Friedberg, Sun, and Webb (2008) analyzed data from the American Time Use Survey and data on retirement from the Health and Retirement Study. The authors found that participation in certain types of nonwork activities is substantially impacted by work. These activities are household activities, leisure activities, and activities of daily living and instrumental activities of daily living, which include eating, sleeping, and grooming. Older people working in jobs in which their leisure activities are limited are more likely to leave those jobs for retirement or to search for new jobs. On the other hand, workers in jobs that impact household activities are less likely to leave their work. Also, those in jobs that have a strong impact on activities such as sleeping, eating, and grooming may be more likely to take new jobs, but are less likely to retire.

The motivation to make the switch from a present occupation to a different one may be the function of the push of a present job and the pull of an alternative career (Feldman, 2007). According to Kahn and Byosiere (1992), job stress is a major push factor related to late-life career change. Feldman, Leana, and Bolina (2002) report that older people, particularly those with financial means, may be more willing to leave highly stressful careers in order to change to more meaningful and less stressful jobs. An occupation-level factor that may motivate an older person to switch careers is the degree of change in skills and work context required to be successful (Hermans & Oles, 1999). Examples of the changes in skill level and work context are the computer proficiency and comfort with social media now required in many careers. While some feel comfortable developing expertise with computers and social media, others feel that the careers they were proficient in have become something different, and they do not want to acquire new skills. As a result of this, they choose to change to another career or job title that may represent the work context they are comfortable in, and more in line with their present skill set.

Johnson, Kawachi, and Lewis (2009) examined the characteristics of the jobs taken by those who re-career. Their research indicates that 3 in 10 late-life career changes follow job layoffs or business closings, and that financial need was an important driver in career change. Although hourly wages are lower for all individuals making a career change, retirees lose the most (approximately 57%). Health benefits are also likely to be lost in the new position. Many of those in new careers move from managerial positions to other areas, such as sales. On the plus side, those in new careers are satisfied in their jobs and report that they have more flexible work schedules and less stress than in their old jobs. Even with the drop in wages and loss of health care coverage, very few of those in the survey making a career change reported disliking their jobs.

Why Reinvent?

People reinvent their work careers for a variety of reasons. In some situations, an individual would like to retire from one career, but would also like to keep working for a while. From a practical perspective, many older people consider new career opportunities in order to maintain financial security. The economic recession in 2008 to 2009 affected many who were planning to retire. While some stayed in their long-term jobs, others retired and looked for other work. Some were either encouraged to retire early or were laid off from their careers. For these individuals, the desire to work at an older age was compounded by the financial insecurity of being without a paycheck. In addition, a 2010 Harris poll indicated that 2% of people 65 and over and 25% of people 46 to 64 have no retirement savings (Harris Interactive, 2010).

Other individuals looking to re-career find work in a different area in order to strengthen their interactions with others. One component of the interpersonal realm is the concept of mattering, developed by Rosenberg and McCullough (1981). *Mattering* is the need to feel noticed, appreciated, and depended upon by others. There are five components of mattering: attention, importance, appreciation, dependence, and pride. Schlossberg (2009) has expanded the concept of mattering to focus on the older person during retirement, stating that older people want to continue to have these mattering connections whether or not their retirement plan continues to include employment. Those looking to explore new career opportunities will look for ones that ensure that they will count in the lives of others (see Chapter 2 for a description of the Purposeful Theory of Aging). For example, someone who retires from a career as a reference librarian may take a part-time job

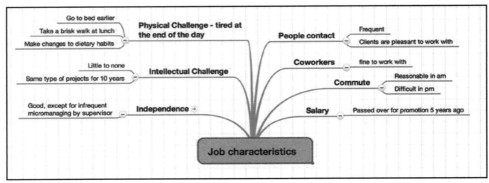

Figure 11-1. Concept map of characteristics of present job.

providing resources on a smoking cessation hotline because it provides a similar connection with others, incorporating the concept of mattering in her work.

Many older people thinking of retirement consider *bridge careers*—employment that takes place after an individual has retired from full-time work, but before one has left the workforce entirely. According to Kim and Feldman (2000) and Cahill, Giandrea, and Quinn (2006), those accepting bridge employment were more likely to be in excellent health, have been in a job for an extended period of time, and had a working spouse and dependent children. Those who were older or had a higher salary were less likely to accept bridge employment, and were more likely to retire completely when leaving their job. The research indicates that bridge employment was strongly correlated to both retirement satisfaction and overall life satisfaction. Cahill et al. (2006) also indicated that current older adults may work longer than the cohort of older people reaching retirement age in the early 1980s. A qualitative study of older workers in the Washington, D.C. area (Ulrich & Brott, 2005) indicates that bridge jobs provide the means to define retirement as a positive opportunity. Those participating in a bridge job viewed retirement as a continuance of their previous life because it incorporated aspects of responsibility, obligations, and choice.

What Am I Looking to Reinvent?

Even before one starts the process to find a new career, it is important to find out what one is trying to change. After being in a career for a long time, it is quite common to view challenges in the workplace as unfixable, and only tolerable in the short term. Part of the preparation for a new career should involve looking at the strengths and weaknesses of one's present career and clarify the problems one is trying to solve by making a career change. Using a tool such as concept mapping (http://www.udel.edu/chem/white/teaching/ConceptMap.html) or mind mapping (Buzan, 1996) is helpful to ensure that all relevant concepts and ideas are considered. While concept mapping was originally developed to help people learn new information, it is also extremely useful in getting a better understanding of a given topic. A concept map or mind map can easily be hand-written on paper. In addition, there are many concept mapping and mind mapping software tools available for computer, tablet and smart phone.

Figure 11-1 is an example of a concept map developed by 66-year-old Jonas, who is trying to decide whether or not he should leave his job of 15 years. As a result of drawing the concept map, Jonas found that he has several areas in which he feels a good deal of job satisfaction, particularly enjoying his relationships with coworkers and clients, and the sense of independence he feels while doing his work.

When asked about it, Jonas says he definitely he feels that he matters in the work environment. However, he does find challenges in the following areas: salary, physical challenge (he is exhausted at the end of the day), a long evening commute, and lack of intellectual challenge. By working further on the concept map, Jonas realistically considers that while his stagnant salary is frustrating, it is ample for his present needs, and given a slow economy, it may not change in the future. He also realizes that he can try to solve his problem with physical exhaustion in a variety of ways: he can make different food choices at breakfast and lunch to see if he will have more energy at the end of the day, he can go to bed at an earlier time, and he can take a short walk at lunch to see if he feels more refreshed. For the long evening commute, Jonas can consider asking his supervisor to change his work schedule slightly so that he can cut his commuting time by 45 minutes each day. After thinking about it further, Jonas realizes that the most frustrating part of his work is the lack of intellectual challenge he has. Jonas has been involved in similar projects for the last 10 years, and is looking to expand his horizons. He plans to spend time determining if leaving his job is the only option, or if he may be able to work out new job responsibilities with his supervisor.

Resources for Reinvention: Finding New Career Ideas

Older people like Jonas understand that reinvention requires developing certain skills. The amount and depth of assistance needed to foster reinvention depends upon several concepts. The first examines how far the new career direction differs from the old. If the individual is tweaking his present career to develop a new one, looking at career resources in the new area, networking with others in the field, and examining general career resources (see Additional Resources at the end of this chapter) may be sufficient. For someone like Jonas, this level of career examination may be sufficient because the change he is looking for is rather limited.

However, if the person is planning to move into a totally different area, more direction may be required. For some, exploring options for new areas of work may be sufficient. Books such as *Great Jobs for Everyone 50+* and *Second-Act Careers* (see Additional Resources) provide information on work opportunities depending on the needs of the job seeker. These books contain information on snowbird jobs, work-at-home jobs, and entrepreneurial opportunities, including what the jobs entail, salary ranges, and the types of people that might enjoy the work.

Others seeking a new career may find that they need to explore a little bit about themselves before making a job switch. For some, this may be necessary because they did not spend time during adulthood exploring their personality, personal goals, and values. Many working adults find they have little time to explore these issues and plan for the future. With aging, those individuals may benefit from self-reflection to find a career that is in line with aspects of their personality. In addition, self-reflection can help avoid career choices that may not have worked for them in the past. For individuals who are happiest exploring options by themselves, books such as *What's Your Type of Career?* and *The Pathfinder: How to Choose or Change Your Career for a Lifetime of Satisfaction and Success* may be useful (see Additional Resources). These books not only explore the nuances of different personality types, but they provide guidance on which careers may be good for a given personality type.

According to Feldman (2007), of the Big Five personality traits often studied in organizational research (Digman, 1989), openness to experience and neuroticism are the most likely to affect career change. Feldman reports, "Older workers who are in good mental health and who have realistic and positive self-regard are also more likely to estimate their chances of success in a new career to be higher as well. Some other personality variables which might be important here are extraversion and self-efficacy" (2007, p. 182). With a lifetime of dealing with change, many adults reach old age with a clear picture of how much change they are able to tolerate. As in earlier adulthood, some people look forward to new experiences, and are ready to try new things. Others are more interested in maintaining the status quo. Regardless of their comfort with novelty, most adults make calculated risks, weighing the pros and cons of a given idea before moving forward. By the time they are ready to make a change, they have prepared well, and are aware that their outcome may or may not be successful.

Other older career changers looking to explore new options may benefit from working with a career counselor. The National Board of Certified Counselors has lists of certified counselors by geographic area. Career counselors on the website also list credentials, desired clientele, testing offered, and specialization, such as career and aging. Contacting a potential career counselor either by phone or email can help the individual understand more about what the career counseling process will entail from time, energy, and financial perspectives.

Another concept the older person needs to consider is the state of his or her health in relation to the physical demands of a job. According to Feldman (2007), the physical requirement of a given job is a greater motivator to change careers for older workers than younger workers. A healthy older person may find it easy to transition to a new career with high physical and cognitive requirements, understanding that the adjustment may take additional time than was required at an earlier age. Someone with multiple, chronic medical conditions with some physical limitations, however, would need to spend added time determining how to overcome the additional challenges required by this new career. While some adaptations are minor and can be handled by the individual or with guidance from friends or family members, others may find it necessary to consult with their primary care physician and get medical clearance to take on new responsibilities. In addition, the career changer may want to consult with an occupational therapist, which can be helpful in making adaptations to the new job setting so that the work will not be overly stressful for the individual.

Which Idea Is Best for Me?

While the first step in the career and work reinvention process is coming up with ideas for new work that are within the ballpark of what is acceptable, the second step in the process involves deciding which is the best choice to pursue. Having criteria to determine the best possible option helps the individual avoid making a decision based on poor or limited reasoning. There are many criteria that can be tailored to the individual needs of a client. For example, one person may look forward to a new career that provides a great deal of intellectual stimulation. An individual who felt mentally taxed by a previous job may want a career that is less intellectually challenging.

Examples of criteria that can be used to evaluate options for reinvention include the following:

- How much training is required to get up to speed in a given career? Does this fit within my expected timeframe for retraining?

- Are there options within my new career area in my geographic location?

- Will my new career require relocation?

- Are there individuals with whom I can network to establish connections and possibly find work?

- Will the option fit my requirements for financial compensation?

- Will I be able to handle the physical challenges of the position/career?

- Will I be able to handle the psychological challenges of the position/career?

- Does the career fit my strengths?

- Will the career meet my requirements for personal contact?

- Will the career provide the appropriate level of intellectual stimulation?

- Will the career allow for flexibility?

- Will the career allow me to achieve my short-term and long-term goals?

- If I am starting a new business, will the outlay required fit within my budget?

Using these criteria to evaluate each career opportunity may help the individual eliminate several options, and he or she may be left with a limited number of choices. At that point, it may be helpful to evaluate each option more carefully, asking the following questions:

- What do I like about career choice A?

- What are some concerns I have with pursuing career choice A?

- What are the opportunities that would emerge from following through on career choice A?

- Are there ways that I can overcome some of my concerns with pursuing career choice A?

Spending time thinking about these questions yields an indepth picture of the benefits and challenges that will take place if a choice is followed. It also helps uncover the barriers and assisters for making a given choice work. For example, someone may really want to pursue a given career, but be concerned by the length of time required to be educated in a new area. By spending time researching how to overcome those concerns, the individual may discover that there is an online program that will cut the training time in half and does not require the half-hour travel each way to the local college.

Making the decision to reinvent and then finding ways to do so can be a challenge no matter what your age. For older people, however, having fewer options may provide an additional challenge. Cara's story demonstrates that no matter the financial and personal challenges one has, satisfying reinvention that incorporates one's passions, interests, and values can occur at any age.

Cara is a tall, striking woman of 79, and according to her, she is on her 8th life already. Cara grew up in upstate New York, and even from a young age, she wanted to be an actress. She also knew that going to college was a remote possibility. Cara married young and said goodbye to her acting career, bur never stopped thinking of a career on the stage. While her marriage was not a good one, she remained in the marriage for quite a while. Eventually, she made the decision to end her marriage when her oldest child married. At that time, her youngest was 14 years of age.

Following her divorce, Cara decided to go to New York City to try to be an actress. When she left, Cara's youngest child remained in upstate New York with her father. During Cara's time in New York, she performed in an off-Broadway play. While Cara got great reviews, she realized that she might not have the personality to handle the actor's life, as auditioning was particularly difficult for her. She had a discussion with friends of her roommate about other career possibilities. One woman working in fashion said that the next big thing in the fashion industry was a high-end store for plus-size women.

When Cara returned to Buffalo a few months later, she decided to open a high-end clothing store for plus-size women, even though she had no experience running a business. She sold her house for cash to open the store. As she said, "so much to be said for stupidity." Without even basic knowledge of business terms or store inventory, she quickly developed the skills to run the store.

The store took off right away, and Cara was extremely successful. Over time, the business grew and she had seven employees, including her sister, daughter, and son. During that time period, Cara reported that she made and spent a lot of money, and many of her customers became her friends. She traveled the world, and bought a house in Spain. Success with the clothing store lasted for 17 years. At that time, Cara reported that many customers stopped buying expensive items. While her accountant suggested that she close the business, Cara poured all her savings into the business so it could stay open for an additional year.

After closing the store at age 65, Cara lived in a rented house. Because she had a niece and nephew in Las Vegas, Cara and her daughter eventually moved to Las Vegas and looked for work. While she was in Las Vegas, she worked in four casinos. Cara remained in Las Vegas for 2 years, purchased a house there, and also found some time to act in a play.

Cara returned to upstate New York in 2000, leaving her house to her daughter in Las Vegas. Back in New York, she found a series of jobs. In one, she worked for the local county government researching welfare fraud, and found that she loved that job. At another job, she worked in disaster relief for the Small Business Administration, helping people who had lost everything. She enjoyed both jobs because she had the opportunity to interact with people and hear their stories. According to Cara, some people are glorious, and some are not. Cara also picked up some theater work when parts were available.

Three and a half years ago, her daughter had a stroke. Cara took a leave from her telemarketing position and flew to Las Vegas to care for her daughter. While there, she sold the house and packed it up to move her daughter back to New York. Cara and her daughter were able to return to New York after 4 months, and she continued to get better there.

Unfortunately, her daughter experienced a second stroke 6 months later, and she died shortly after. Cara stated that this was a very difficult period in her life. She said that one needs to make friends with the grief and it becomes a way of being.

Following the death of her daughter, Cara began work at her local senior center. She continues to work there, doing anything they need her to do, such as working in the gift shop or café, or helping out in the dining room. Cara reports that she likes the contact with people. In addition, she has delivered meals for the agency. Cara still does some theater work, and recently played the part of a priest's housekeeper. Cara meditates, does yoga, and reports that her energy level has decreased with age.

When Cara was asked about reinvention, she said that it "changes your life in a very meaningful way. The idea is to find something during the reinvention process to change your life into something that is meaningful and you enjoy." In the last few months, Cara has started to take classes in hopes of doing voiceover work in commercials and books on tape. Cara has a beautiful speaking voice, and she hopes that her work will become consistent because she wants to create a steady stream of income. She also said that she does not have a step-by-step plan for the future. Instead, she allows things to percolate, knowing that something of interest will come along that will allow her to incorporate both her love of acting and working with people.

Cara is an example of an older person who has had several changes in employment since the age of 65. She has taken opportunities to reinvent herself in relation to work and has drawn on her many years of skills and experience in a variety of settings. A number of these career changes, such as working for disaster relief and at her local senior center, encompass the concept of "mattering" referred to earlier in this chapter. All have provided her with quality of life and well-being.

CONCLUSION

This chapter has described retirement as a catalyst for a new beginning in how older people choose to spend their energy. Retirement may open eligibility, ideas, and opportunities for new employment adventures. The concepts discussed in this chapter are reflected throughout the book by people who told their stories, such as Catherine and Rachel in Chapter 2. Many older people need ongoing career goals to explore once they retire from a current career, and many dream of turning those hobbies into new employment. Finally, the continued need to be purposeful and to continue to matter to others often brings older people back into employment, and proves to be energizing and motivating.

REFERENCES

Alzheimer's Society. (2013). Retrieved May 7, 2013, from http://dementiacatalogue.alzheimers.org.uk/library/library-Home.do.

Australian Human Rights Commission. (2008). Retrieved May 7, 2013, from http://www.humanrights.gov.au/publications/mature-workers-case-studies-workplace#1_1.

Buzan, T., & Buzan, B. (1996). *The mind map book: How to use radiant thinking to map your brain's untapped potential.* New York, NY: Plume.

Cahill, K. E., Giandrea, M. D., & Quinn, J. F. (2006). Retirement patterns from career employment. *The Gerontologist, 46,* 514-523.

Digman, J. M. (1989). Five robust trait dimensions: Development, stability, and utility. *Journal of Personality, 57,* 195-214.

Feldman, D. C. (2002). Second careers and multiple careers. In R. J. Burke & C. L. Cooper (Eds.), *The new world of work* (pp. 75-94). Oxford, UK: Blackwell.

Feldman, D. C. (2007). Career mobility and career stability among older workers. In K. S. Shultz & G. A. Adams (Eds.), *Aging and work in the 21st century* (pp. 179-197). Mahwah, NJ: Lawrence Erlbaum Associates.

Feldman, D. C., Leana, C. R., & Bolino, M. (2002). Underemployment among downsized executives: Test of a mediated effects model. *Journal of Occupational and Organizational Psychology, 75,* 453-471.

Freedman, M. (2008). *Encore: Finding work that matters in the second half of life.* New York, NY: Public Affairs.

Friedberg, L., Sun, W., & Webb, A. (2008). What effects do time constraints have on the age of retirement? *Center for Retirement Research at Boston College.* Retrieved from https://www2.bc.edu/~sunwc/paper/2008-17.pdf.

Harris Interactive (2010) retrieved May 7, 2013, from http://www.harrisinteractive.com/NewsRoom/HarrisPolls/tabid/447/mid/1508/articleId/684/ctl/ReadCustom%20Default/Default.aspx.

Hermans, H. J. M., & Oles, P. K. (1999). Midlife crisis in men: Affective organization of personal meanings. *Human Relations, 52*(11), 1403-1426.

Johnson, R. W., Kawachi, J., & Lewis, E. K. (2009). *Older adults on the move: Recareering in later life.* AARP Public Policy Institute. Retrieved May 7, 2013, from www.urban.org/uploadedpdf/1001272_olderworksonthmove.pdf.

Kahn, R. L., & Byosiere, P. (1992). Stress in organizations. In M. D. Dunnette & L. M. Hough (Eds.), *Handbook of industrial and organizational psychology* (2nd ed., Vol. 3, pp. 571-650). Palo Alto, CA: Consulting Psychologists Press.

Kim, S., & Feldman, D. C. (2000). Working in retirement: The antecedents of bridge employment and its consequences for quality of life in retirement. *Academy of Management Journal, 43,* 1195-1210.

Reinvention [Def. 3]. (n.d.). *dictionary.com.* Retrieved January 2, 2013, from http://dictionary.reference.com/browse/reinvention?s=t.

Rosenberg, M., & McCullough, B. C. (1981). Mattering: Inferred significance to parents and mental health among adolescents. In R. Simmons (Ed.), *Research in Community and Mental Health* (pp. 163-182). Greenwich, CT: JAI Press.

Schlossberg, N. K. (2009). *Revitalizing retirement: Reshaping your identity, relationships, and purpose.* Washington, DC: American Psychological Association.

Ullman, S. (n.d.). Youth. *UAB—Samuel Ullman Museum—Home.* Retrieved June 6, 2014, from http://www.uab.edu/ullmanmuseum/.

Ulrich, L. B., & Brott, P. E. (2005). Older workers and bridge employment: Redefining retirement. *Journal of Employment Counseling, 43*(4), 159-170.

ADDITIONAL RESOURCES

Books

Collamer, N. (2013). *Second-act career: 50+ ways to profit from your passions during semi-retirement.* Berkeley, CA: Ten Speed Press.

Corbett, D., & Higgins, R. (2006). *Portfolio life: The new path to work, purpose and passion after 50.* San Francisco, CA: Jossey-Bass.

Dunning, D. (2010). *What's your type of career?* (2nd Ed.). Boston: Nicholas Brealey Publishing.

Epstein, L. (2007). *Working after retirement for dummies.* Hoboken, NJ: John Wiley and Sons.

Freedman, M. (2008). *Encore: Finding work that matters in the second half of life.* New York, NY: Public Affairs.

Freedman, M. (2011). *The big shift: Navigating the new stage beyond midlife.* New York, NY: Public Affairs.

Hannon, K. (2012). *Great jobs for everyone 50+: Finding work that keeps you happy and healthy and pays the bills.* Hoboken: John Wiley & Sons, Inc.

Lore, N. (2011). *The pathfinder: How to choose or change your career for a lifetime of satisfaction and success* (Rev. ed,). New York, NY: Touchstone

Schlossberg, N. K. (2009). *Revitalizing retirement: Reshaping your Identity, relationships, and purpose.* Washington, D.C.: American Psychological Association.

Sedlar, J., & Miners, R. (2007). *Don't retire, rewire* (2nd Ed.). New York, NY: ALPHA.

Tieger, P., & Barron-Tieger, B. (2007). *Do what you are: Discover the perfect career through the secrets of personality type* (4th ed.). Boston: Little, Brown and Company.

Websites

AARP: Resources for work as an older adult. http://www.aarp.org/work/

About.com: Career planning after retirement. http://careerplanning.about.com/od/diversityresources/a/retirement.htm

Forbes: The Forbes Retirement Guide. http://www.forbes.com/special-report/2011/03/23/retirement-guide.html

Kiplinger: Resources for work after retirement. http://www.kiplinger.com/features/archives/2008/07/rpg_resources_for_work_after_retirement.html

National Board of Certified Counselors: http://www.nbcc.org/counselorfind

Rockport Institute: Resources for developing a new career path. http://www.rockportinstitute.com/

U.S. Department of Labor Job Loss Resources: Health and retirement benefits after job loss http://www.dol.gov/ebsa/publications/joblosstoolkit.html#.UMIcXI5S3qE

Your Encore: A website to match life science, consumer products, and food industries with recently retired experts. http://www.yourencore.com/

12

Sustainability

Caroline Wolverson, DipCOT, DipHT, MSc and
Linda A. Hunt, PhD, OTR/L, FAOTA

I've decided to pick my moment to retire very carefully—in about 200 years' time.—Brian Clough (Powell, 2010)

Currently, there is increasing recognition not only of the needs of older people, but also of what they are able to continue to contribute to society. Maintaining productive engagement as people enter old age has the potential to improve well-being and extend working lives, and through this provide a stimulus for economic growth, reducing the overall strain on health and social care systems (Eurostat, 2011). Until recently, retirement has perhaps been promoted as a state of reward for years of work, with time to enjoy and focus on previous ambitions that have not been realized (Balandin, Llewellyn, Dew, Ballin, & Schneider, 2006). Given current financial pressures, this view is idealistic. Continued adequate job performance is the necessary condition for remaining in employment. Fitness for the job role is evaluated on workers' health, function, knowledge, and skills, the requirements of the job, and the signals from employer and coworkers about the value of an individual's efforts. A key concept is that of *active aging*, which came into prominence during the United Nations Year of Older People 1999; it involves harnessing the skills and talents of older people (Hunter, 2011). It recognizes that if people are working longer, they need to maintain a good level of health and well-being, with access to healthy workplaces, flexible working, lifelong learning, and retirement plans (Eurostat, 2011).

This chapter considers how government, organizational, and community initiatives, along with private companies, can address some of the challenges facing older people remaining in the workforce, and support them in maintaining a productive lifestyle. It will suggest ways to capitalize on and sustain the skills and resources of older people by providing an enabling and supportive society in which they can continue to flourish.

The World Health Organization (WHO) (2007) refers to older people as a resource for their families, communities, and the economy, while recognizing that they need supportive and enabling living environments to achieve this. When working past traditional retirement ages,

- 135 -

Hunt LA, Wolverson C.
Work and the Older Person: Increasing Longevity and Well-Being (pp 135-145).
© 2015 SLACK Incorporated.

older people and society must undergo a change in perception and attitude. Of course, not all older people benefit from continued employment, so choice is essential. Ekerdt (2010) writes that retirement may be a developmental need or a response to cultural suggestion, and provides a historical overview of how scholars viewed retirement. Elon Moore (1946) wrote that retirement can be a fulfilling time of life if retirees remain active and socially engaged: "Many studies attest to the fact that the greatest unhappiness comes from the lack of busy-ness" (p. 209). Retirement can have an impact on identity, roles (Pettican & Prior, 2011), and social status (Price, 2002). As long ago as 1947, Nathan Shock wrote a ringing defense of the performance potential of older workers. He marshaled research findings to rebut the contention that older workers had increased labor turnover, accident rates, illness, and absenteeism. Even when diminished function is likely, employers can accommodate older workers, particularly in today's society where there is access to such a vast range of technology. Shock concluded, "The rapid increase in the proportion of older individuals in our society makes it imperative that plans be made for utilizing the capabilities of the older worker in our national economy" (p. 101). Ewan Clague (1949) brought life span and work span projections from the U.S. Department of Labor to bear on the question of whether increased life expectancy in coming decades would be spent in or out of the labor force. Through our interviews with aging individuals for this book, we found that continued employment and/or volunteer work brought purpose and greater quality of life for older people. Many reported they were healthy enough to continue working well past the traditional retirement age of 60-plus years. Many had no plans for retirement, and saw part-time work in their future as they aged. Some felt that they complemented a younger workforce with their drive for excellence, knowledge, and commitment to learn new information, therefore sustaining the longevity of an aging workforce.

Government Responses to an Aging Population

Governments are continuing to focus on the older population and are giving high priority to extending working lives. The year 2012 was designated that of "Active ageing and solidarity between generations" by the European Union. The U.S. Department of Health and Human Services has made the well-being of older people a priority in the national *Healthy People 2020 Framework* (2010), with a focus on improving health, function, and quality of life. In the United Kingdom, the Department of Work and Pensions developed a 2-year "Aging Well" program. This program came to an end in 2012, but its legacy continues within the local areas that were targeted and good practice examples are available for others to follow. Documents such as *Employing Older Workers: An Employer's Guide to Today's Multigenerational Workforce* (Department of Work and Pensions, 2013) offer support for businesses to maintain an older workforce. Despite this, *Ready for Ageing*, a report by the UK House of Lords select committee (2012), highlighted that they were disappointed to see how little the UK government had done to initiate a long-term strategy to deal with the consequence of an aging population. They confirmed the need for older people to be offered flexible retirement in the form of part-time work, while administering pensions, benefits, and tax relief in a more flexible way. In 2011, the compulsory retirement age of 65 was abolished in the United Kingdom and the state pension age will rise to 67 by 2028; ministers have warned that they are unsure of pension ages in the future (*Gerontology News*, 2013).

An article by Meyer (2013) reported on a policy review in the United Kingdom of European initiatives to support longer working lives. This recognizes the need for the United Kingdom to implement more effective strategies to keep older people in work. Some good practice examples highlighted are in Sweden (where subsidies are offered to employers who recruit older workers on long-term contracts), and Germany (whose government intends to offer increased flexibility and more options for sabbaticals for older workers).

In recognizing that the United Kingdom's future economic success is dependent on the skills and contributions of older workers, the minister for higher education has suggested that older workers who continue their education will maintain their skills, and as a result, they will be more likely to remain employed. To support this, the age limit on student loans (including tuition fees) has been lifted. However, advocates for older people are unsure if they will be able, or willing, to enroll and commit to challenging coursework, along with increased debt, to continue working (*Gerontology News*, 2013).

Change is also taking place in Canada. An article published in 2013 reported that the Canadian federal government will begin to increase the age of eligibility from 65 to 67 for old age security and guaranteed income supplement payments in 2023 (*Gerontology News*, 2013). A recent study by the Bank of Montreal of 1,000 Canadians aged 18 years and over found that 81% plan on doing some kind of work in their retirement years; two reasons were as a hobby, and to "stay sharp." The survey revealed that 40% reported that they were likely to start their own business during retirement. Nearly half of respondents indicated that they would use some of their retirement savings to fund their business (*Gerontology News*, 2013).

France is seeking pension reform because the large aging population has exacerbated the vulnerability of the French system. It has proved difficult to reduce the early exit of older workers from the labor market. Beland and Durandal (2013) wrote a compelling overview of aging in France highlighting issues regarding retirement policy and pension funds. Currently, on average, both men and women exit the labor market at age 59. Postponing the average retirement age has long been a key policy challenge in France. Before a major reform that took place in 1993, workers had to contribute for only 37.5 years in total to qualify for regular public pension benefits. In 2012, this number stood at 41 years. As for public-sector workers, a major reform enacted in 2003 reduced the gap between their pensions and the ones available to private-sector workers, and homogenized the duration of the required contribution period to reach eligibility for a full pension. In 2010, a new pension reform was established to increase the minimum eligibility age gradually from 60 to 62. Following the May 2012 presidential election, however, the new Socialist government announced a series of measures allowing workers who began their career before age 20 and had contributed to the program for at least 41.5 years to retire with full benefits at 60. Education about active and healthy aging through staying employed may be needed in France.

CHALLENGES TO CONTINUED WORKING

There are a number of challenges that make it more difficult for older people to continue to work. A study by the Equality & Human Rights Commission (2010) carried out a telephone survey with 1,500 people aged 50 to 75 about their working lives and aspirations. The study also reviewed employer practices and interviewed interested parties, such as government, trade unions, and nonprofit organizations. Key barriers to continued work were poor health, lack of flexibility and choice, employers' attitudes toward older workers, and work dissatisfaction. Further barriers may be the lack of the key characteristics for "age-friendly cities" as identified by the WHO (2007), such as respect and social inclusion, transportation, and the built environment.

MAINTAINING A PRODUCTIVE LIFESTYLE WITH DECLINING HEALTH: ADAPTIVE APPROACHES

Poor health is perceived as a key driver in early retirement, and as such, maintaining independence is increasingly important to keep older people working, contributing to economic growth, and reducing strain on health and social services (Eurostat, 2011). Older disabled workers or those with health issues should not be excluded from maintaining a productive lifestyle (see Chapter 4). Evidence shows they have less opportunity and are often excluded from the workforce. In the United

Kingdom, supported employment opportunities such as REMPLOY (http://www.remploy.co.uk/) continue to be marginalized as the government closes down these work environments. This exclusion from a productive lifestyle is likely to increase as the older person reaches retirement; disadvantaged both by disability and age. For disabled workers, the roles and opportunities offered by the workplace may hold greater significance because they may experience more social isolation in their home lives than nondisabled workers. Consequently, their social isolation will become more significant once they are no longer working (Balandin, Llewellyn, Dew, Ballin, & Schneider, 2006). Although appropriate retirement planning may still be sparse for the nondisabled worker, Balandin et al. (2006) suggest that in supported employment, there may also be a lack of preretirement planning, further compounding the challenges that older disabled workers may face in maintaining a productive lifestyle beyond retirement.

Older people should consider opportunities for retraining in order to keep up to date with technological advances. Although this might be a challenge, these technological advances can help workers remain in the workplace by providing adapted environments and ways of continuing to meet the demands of the job (see Chapter 10).

Maximizing occupational performance requires consideration of the dynamic interaction between the person, the occupation, and the environment. Diane's story illustrates how adaptation of the social environment and the occupation can facilitate continued engagement:

> *Diane was diagnosed with early-onset dementia at the age of 59. She had to take early retirement from her job as a factory worker, which she had held for over 30 years. She felt that her life no longer had focus or purpose, and she missed the social contact and camaraderie of the workplace. In addition to the challenges caused by her diagnosis, her mental well-being began to decline. Given her remaining skills, it was determined that Diane could make a contribution as a volunteer at a day service for people with dementia. She was able to take on a productive role, helping to provide refreshments, clear tables, clean up, and help other staff with group activities. The skilled staff at the day service were able to provide support at just the right level to enable Diane to succeed and make a valuable contribution. Occupations were adapted to ensure success. Diane and her family recognized that as her condition progressed, she would need the services of the adult day care center, but by working as a volunteer, the transition would be eased because the environment and staff would be familiar to her. This supportive environment provided Diane with a flexible way to maintain a productive lifestyle that had been so necessary to her sense of self throughout her working life.*

The physical environment can also have a detrimental effect on health, or exacerbate existing poor health. The principles of inclusive design (called universal design in the United States), should be considered to maximize health and well-being. This approach to design ensures that products and services meet the needs of the widest possible audience, regardless of age and ability (Design Council, 2013).

A further consideration for those experiencing injury, illness, or an acquired disability should be opportunity for rehabilitation. This is an area of potential prejudice for the older person. Frequently, the goal of rehabilitation is for them to return home or remain in their home with the focus on independence in daily living tasks. Governments and service providers need to recognize that this may meet the physical needs of the person, but neglect the psychological and social needs. Reablement services (Social Care Institute for Excellence, 2013), are beginning to recognize this, and while this report does not specifically refer to the older person returning to work, it does highlight the importance of psychological and social needs being met. A key factor of satisfactory rehabilitation is an integrated relationship between health and social services, alongside community resources. A broader approach should be taken that is not limited by prejudicial expectations of what an older person's lifestyle should be.

RETIREMENT PLANNING

With increasing longevity, a much larger number of people will be experiencing retirement for a longer period of time. Planning for this life stage by the individual, and support from employers and society, will assist in maintaining health and well-being. A study by Taylor and Doverspike (2003) highlighted that retirement planning is of critical importance to personal and economic well-being in old age, yet evidence suggests that people are frequently unprepared. Adams and Rau (2011) refer to the importance of self-regulation and monitoring; continually revising expectations both before and during retirement. In their study exploring the occupational transition of retirement, Pettican and Prior (2011) found a close, multifaceted link between occupational engagement and the maintenance of health and well-being. Andonian and MacRae (2011) researched strategies to maintaining social participation for older people within an urban environment and found that, for some, opportunity for successful social participation required effort, energy, and planning. Remaining in employment provides ready-made opportunities for social participation.

The lack of flexibility, choice of hours, and location were highlighted as barriers to continued employment in the Equality and Human Rights Commission study (2010). Opportunities for *bridge employment* may help to address this. Quinn (2002) defines bridge employment as "part-time or short-duration jobs that occur between full-time career employment and complete labor force withdrawal" (p. 295). Bridge employment may offer the opportunity to work fewer hours, have less stress and responsibility, as well as greater flexibility and fewer physical demands in the workplace (Feldman, 1994). This can be advantageous to the employer, who can utilize the skills and knowledge of the older worker, and to the individual, who is able to maintain some income while preparing for and adjusting to full retirement. Mrs. Rogers can be considered a successful example of bridge employment:

> *Mrs. Rogers worked for 37 years in banking. She retired at age 71 and returned to work at 72. Her skill set—specialization in home mortgage lending—was valued, and so she was invited to work part-time in that area. Widowed at a young age, Mrs. Rogers "went back to work full-time when my twins were 5 years old. Socially, I gravitated towards other women who were in the work world. I still see people who worked with me. I keep in touch with some on a regular basis. All of my old friends were not made in the workplace. I have friends from when I was 5 years old."*
>
> *When asked how this part-time work differs from her full-time work responsibilities, Mrs. Rogers stated: "Being able to get going with the day. That is one thing that I enjoy. What I like is taking my time. Having coffee, checking the news. Letting the day unfold. I like this more relaxed style. I know people who are retired and I do not see them losing interest in the world. Some people are happy if they are productive. Everybody is different. My full-time job changed from salary to commission. Ethically, I could not handle that. I did not want my best performance based on commission. That big change made me decide to retire. Everyone told me that when it is time to retire, you will know."*

Many older people view retirement as a means to gain a sense of freedom and control in their lives. It does not necessarily follow that they want to stop working. Financial security offers a means to pursue long-held ambitions, to take work in a new direction. In her article for the *Wall Street Journal*, Essick (2012) spoke to Gerald Leemer, who had worked for 35 years as an accountant, including 25 years as a partner in the firm. He had reached the point financially where he was able to retire. He now volunteers for five shifts a month as an emergency medical technician. Although this has involved intensive training, it brings many rewards, including providing both physical and cognitive challenges. Leemer states:

> *Accounting was very intellectual. Now my job is emotional and physical and requires split-second reaction.*

I didn't just quit overnight. I white-boarded my goal, listing all my requirements for my next act: no set schedule, spend time with people, be outdoors, help others, and give back to my community. It was fantastic becoming part of a new community and meeting people from all walks of life. Driving an ambulance through congested city streets takes a lot of mental focus and honed reflexes, plus we have to memorize all the area streets with no GPS. (para. 4, 7, 9)

Leemer demonstrates the process of successful aging (Freund, 2008). He is functioning at a level that has enabled him to strive to achieve personal goals and maintain personal standards by having successfully managed both internal and external resources throughout his life span. Freund and Riediger (2001) describe resources as "the means of achieving one's goals." With increasing age, the number of resources an individual can access may be reduced and those present may be drawn upon more extensively. This imbalance may result in unsuccessful aging.

SUPPORTIVE EMPLOYERS

Key to enabling older people to work is a supportive employer. The Equality and Human Rights Commission (2010) highlighted the importance of workplace solutions in maintaining older people in employment. Their study found there were concerns about the negative attitudes of employers—either real or perceived—to employing older workers. Seventy-nine percent of retired people felt that more openness to recruiting older workers would help them to gain employment. The report recommended that government should consider incentives for employers in enabling all workers to have greater flexibility. Training for employers, such as the e-learning age awareness program offered by many companies, can help managers and employers recognize the value of the older workers. A further area of development that larger employers should consider is ensuring that occupational health departments are trained and equipped to support the needs of older workers.

The Age Positive initiative developed by the Department of Work & Pensions in the United Kingdom offers advice and information to employers on managing a multigenerational workforce (2013). The website (https://www.gov.uk/government/organisations/department-for-work-pensions/series/age-positive) also gives case study examples of both employers and employees, such as that of David Buckley.

David Buckley, a sales manager for a textile company, was made redundant at age 60 and spent 9 months on Job Seeker's Allowance, facing rejection after rejection from employers. "Nobody wanted a 60-year-old until Domestic & General came along," he says. He was hired at the company's call center and has worked there ever since. [Now 77] he is the outbound call handler for the heating team, calling customers who need advice, and taking "brickbats and compliments." He says younger colleagues approach him for assistance because of his experience. "I don't feel like an old man. I feel like a person who takes pleasure in work for its own sake." The company uses "age-positive" strategies to attract and keep older workers for their experience, reliability, and loyalty. It targets specific media for hiring, e.g., using radio stations aimed at older listeners. Other strategies include telephone interviews to avoid bias at the first stage of hiring; tailored induction, with extra support in areas such as IT skills; career progression workshops; and flexible work arrangements available to all. The company has no mandatory retirement age, and Mr. Buckley opted to continue working when he reached 65. "I like to feel that I'm part of working life, rather than vegetating. The financial motivation was tremendously important when I was 60. Now the money and having a reason to stay alive are equally important." (Equality & Human Rights Commission, 2010, p. 12)

B&Q, a large retail employer, was the first company in the United Kingdom to target older workers. Approximately a quarter of the workforce is over 50, and their employees range from 16 to 96 years old. Other companies are following this trend, and looking at ways to support the older worker in continued employment.

TRANSPORTATION

Several chapters in this book have highlighted the challenges of transportation for older people. Sustaining the productivity of an individual needs to be considered more broadly than an enabling work environment, but also the support systems surrounding the person. Increasing age brings increasing likelihood of failing eyesight and disability; as a result, the person may no longer be able to drive. If this prevents the person from getting to and from work, the impact on well-being may be significant. Studies by Gustafsson et al. (2011) and Liddle, Gustafsson, Bartlett, and McKenna (2012) found that giving up driving for older people was associated with decreased feelings of control and loss of meaningful roles and occupations. In the United Kingdom, older people are entitled to a free bus pass, which they can use anywhere in the country. This would help the older worker to get to work, from a practical as well as a financial point of view. A further challenge is the increasing isolation of people living in rural communities where local schools, shops, restaurants, and post offices that would have been a source of employment are being closed down. An adequate infrastructure is needed to support older people and communities in general, as highlighted in the WHO's *Global Age-Friendly Cities* (2007).

INTERGENERATIONAL SUPPORT

"Social capital is a concept that highlights relationships within society through the promotion of cooperation; it is often seen as a collectively generated public good derived from the activities of communities and social networks" (Eurostat, 2011, p. 111). This can be applied to the concept of cross-generational support in enabling older people to continue to be fulfilled through work. The focus on intergenerational support to sustain a productive lifestyle for older people is supported by the European Union through the year of "Active ageing and solidarity between generations" (Eurostat, 2011), "however, there appear to be few opportunities for old and young people to meet and exchange ideas in modern societies. Almost-two thirds (63.8%) of the EU-27 population (aged 15 and above) questioned in March 2009 agreed that there were not enough opportunities for older and younger people to meet and work together in associations and local community initiatives" (p. 112).

The examples below illustrate opportunities that have been taken by younger and older generations to work together to enrich their lives and those of others while forging new careers:

> *At the age of 94, Barbara "Cutie" Cooper has developed a role for herself as an "agony aunt," giving relationship advice via an online blog that she set up with the help of her two grand-daughters (Qureshi, 2012). Barbara, who lives in Los Angeles, has also published a book called* Fall in Love for Life. *Her positive approach to life and loss can be summed up in her statement, "Never count yourself out. Every person has something to give, some love or some wisdom or a shoulder to cry upon. As long as you care about others you have a reason to be on this earth. So go take your place in the grand scheme and live your life with all your heart." (Cooper, 2012)*

Barbara's blog can be accessed at http://www.goodreads.com/author/show/6456818. Barbara_Cutie_Cooper/blog.

Beryl Renwick (86) and Betty Smith (90) forged a radio career for themselves by chance:

Beryl and Betty have copresented a weekly radio show for the past 6 years alongside David Reeves, who at 35 is able to complement the pair and "twiddle the knobs," as Betty says. Their local fame on Radio Humberside became national stardom in 2012 when they won Gold at the Sony Awards. Their opportunity came about serendipitously when they went on a tour of the radio station with their local social club, charming their copresenter and giving him the idea for the show. (Williams, 2012)

Both of these examples demonstrate the value of cross-generational links, and how opportunities can be given to older people, and in turn, their skills can be valued by younger generations. They acknowledge the wisdom and experience of the older person, while using the practical skills of the younger person to achieve a goal. The recognition of transferring skills is also provided in the case studies for businesses presented by the Department of Work and Pensions (2013):

Brian joined A. T. Brown Coaches at age 57 as a full-time garage manager. With 50 years' experience, Brian, now 67, plans to continue working part-time rather than retire. When he considered working differently, he discussed options with his manager. A gradual 12-month handover was arranged, and he has moved from full-time to 3 days a week. Brian is mentoring Andy (31) in the garage manager role, where Andy is "learning the lifetime of skills and knowledge they don't teach you in a course!" (p. 15)

A survey conducted in 2011 asked Europeans their opinion of the relative merits of the workforce aged 55 and over. Results suggested that those 55 and over had a somewhat higher opinion of their own qualities in the workplace than the population as a whole, but there was broad agreement on their main traits: experienced, reliable, could make decisions on their own. However, they were not so flexible, open to new ideas, or up-to-date with technology (Eurostat, 2011, p. 53).

RESOURCES TO SUPPORT THE OLDER WORKER

There are a number of other organizations in the United Kingdom that support the older worker and employers: The Intergenerational Foundation (http://www.if.org.uk/) has been established to research fairness between generations, and has a blog discussion that people can engage in. The International Longevity Centre (http://www.ilcuk.org.uk/) is the leading independent think tank on longevity and demographic change. The Age and Employment Network (TAEN) (http://www.taen.org.uk/) works to provide an effective labor market, servicing the needs of those in mid and late life alongside employers and the economy. The charity Grandparents Plus (http://www.grandparentsplus.org.uk/) champions the essential role of grandparents and the wider family in the lives of children. With an increasing number of older people considering alternative work options, The Prince's Initiative for Mature Enterprise (http://www.prime.org.uk/who-we-are/), established by the Prince of Wales, is the only national organization in the United Kingdom that is dedicated to providing everyone over 50, who is unemployed or under threat of redundancy, with the support to achieve financial, social, and personal fulfillment through sustainable self-employment. All these resources offer advice to the individual, and often to employers, about ways of sustaining employment for those moving toward old age.

MAINTAINING A PRODUCTIVE LIFESTYLE BEYOND RETIREMENT

Continued lifelong learning can offer opportunities to maintain a productive lifestyle. In 2009, the British government produced a white paper called *The Learning Revolution*, which set out plans for lifelong learning opportunities. It recognizes that building a culture of learning can help people to adjust to change, increase their self-esteem, develop resilience, and have the confidence to respond to challenges. It can also foster more socially inclusive communities (Department of Innovation, Universities and Skills, 2009). If the concept of lifelong learning is fostered from a young age, it is likely that when reaching older age, the person will continue to see this as a positive option for productive occupation.

The University of the Third Age (U3A) celebrated its 30th anniversary in 2012, offering education as well as creative and leisure opportunities to older people no longer in full-time work. It draws on the knowledge, experience and skills of its members. In the United Kingdom, over 300 subjects are offered. It is a self-help, self-managed learning cooperative. The organization empowers older people to continue with lifelong learning, which can contribute to maintaining self-esteem, health, and well-being. Testimonials from those involved give positive feedback; Terry states: "The U3A has given me confidence to undertake tasks which previously I would not even have considered, and through this wonderful organization I have made three very good friends who I would not otherwise have met" (Member's comments, n.d.).

Another example of shared learning is a relatively recent project called The Amazings (http://www.theamazings.com/). This offers a wide range of informal classes and courses taught in a range of venues, including online. Teachers are people over 50 who have a passion for their subject. Their informative website motto is "Wisdom is the greatest natural resource we have. Let's pass it on." Their vision is "a marketplace for wisdom."

Continuing to share skills to the benefit of others in a low-pressure environment, such as those offered by the U3A and The Amazings, is a clear way of maintaining quality of life and well-being through productivity.

CONCLUSION

The challenges faced by the aging population, and by society adjusting to the change in demographics, are significant but not insurmountable. Continued participation of older people should be seen as the norm in today's society. Not only should we provide opportunities for this, we should recognize the worth of the older person and put it to good use. The change in employment patterns for older people is gaining momentum. Promoting healthy behaviors through the lifespan, and creating physical and social environments to foster health and participation for older people (WHO, 2012), should be the goal of organizations as well as individuals. In Western culture, despite government rhetoric, the reality is that older people are still marginalized, with the focus remaining on youth and the qualities that accompany this (Featherstone & Hepworth, 2005). Dated patterns of thinking about aging can limit society's capacity to identify real challenges presented by aging communities and create opportunities. One of the main goals of the European year of Active Ageing and Solidarity between Generations (Eurostat, 2011) was to challenge the idea that older people are a burden to society. The WHO (2012) suggests that new models of aging should be developed to support these changes. The Theory of Purposeful Aging, introduced in Chapter 3, is an example of this.

A variety of mechanisms have been used around the world to address barriers to the labor market for older people: laws and regulations, tailored interventions, vocational rehabilitation and training, self-employment and microfinance, social protection, and working to change attitudes (WHO, 2011). Implementation of these will hopefully sustain an active older workforce.

REFERENCES

Adams, G. A., & Rau, B. L. (2011). Putting off tomorrow to do what you want today. Planning for retirement. *American Psychologist, 66*(3), 180-192.

Andonian, L., & MacRae, M. (2011). Well older adults within an urban context: Strategies to create and maintain social participation. *British Journal of Occupational Therapy, 74*(1), 2-11.

Balandin, S., Llewellyn, G., Dew, A., Ballin, L. & Schneider, J. (2006). Older disabled workers' perceptions of volunteering. *Disability & Society, 21*(7), 677-692.

Beland, D., & Durandal, J. P. V. (2013). Aging in France: Population trends, policy issues, and research institutions. *The Gerontologist, 53*(2), 191-197.

Clague, E. (1949). Productivity, employment, and living standards. *Bureau of Labor Statistics.* Retrieved July 4, 2013, from http://content.cdlib.org/ark:/28722/bk0004016d/?layout=metadata.

Cooper, B. (2012). *Fall in love for life.* San Francisco, CA: Chronicle Books.

Department of Innovation, Universities and Skills. (2009). *The learning revolution.* Retrieved August 28, 2013, from http://www.bis.gov.uk/assets/BISCore/corporate/MigratedD/publications/L/learning_revolution.pdf.

Department of Work and Pensions. (2013). *Employing older workers: An employer's guide to today's multi-generational workforce.* Retrieved July 2, 2013, from https://www.gov.uk/government/publications/employing-older-workers-an-employer-s-guide-to-today-s-multi-generational-workforce.

Design Council. (2013). *Inclusive design education resource.* Retrieved July 4, 2013, from http://www.designcouncil.info/inclusivedesignresource/index.html.

Ekerdt, D. J. (2010). Frontiers of research on work and retirement. *Journal of Gerontology: Social Sciences, 65B*(1), 69-80.

Equality & Human Rights Commission. (2010) *Working Better The over 50s, the newwork generation.* Retrieved July 7, 2013 from http://www.equalityhumanrights.com/uploaded_files/publications/workingbetter_over_50s.pdf.

Essick, K. (2012). An ex-CPA finds a new life in saving others. *Wall Street Journal* [electronic version] October 22, 2012. Retrieved August 30, 2013, from http://online.wsj.com/article/SB10000872396390443696660457764585080 5288704.html.

Eurostat European Commission. (2011). Active ageing and solidarity between generations: A statistical portrait of the European Union. Retrieved August 28, 2013, from http://epp.eurostat.ec.europa.eu/cache/ITY_OFFPUB/KS-EP-11-001/EN/KS-EP-11-001-EN.PDF.

Featherstone, M., & Hepworth, M. (2005). Images of ageing: Cultural represenations of later life. In M. L. Johnson, V. L. Bengtson, P. G. Coleman, & T. B. L. Kirkwood (Eds.), *The Cambridge handbook of age and ageing.* Cambridge, MA: Cambridge University Press.

Feldman, D. C. (1994). The decision to retire early: A review and conceptualization. *The Academy of Management Review, 19,* 285-311.

Freund, A. M. (2008). Successful aging as management of resources: The role of selection, optimization, and compensation. *Research in Human Development, 5*(2), 94-106.

Freund, A. M., & Riediger, M. (2001). What I have and what I do: The role of resource loss and gain throughout life. *Applied Psychology: An International Review, 50,* 370-380.

Gerontology News. (2013). Britain encourages older adults to return to the classroom. Retrieved April 29, 2013 from http://www.geron.org/images/stories/newsletters/gerontology_news/April_2013.pdf

Gustafsson, L. A., Liddle, J. M., Lua, S., Hoyle, M. F., Pachana, N. A., Mitchell, G. K., & McKenna, K. T. (2011). Participant feedback and satisfaction with the UQDRIVE groups for driving cessation. *Canadian Journal of Occupational Therapy, 78*(2), 110-117.

House of Lords Select Committee on Public Service and Demographic Change. (2013). *Ready for Ageing?* Retrieved July 2, 2013, from http://www.publications.parliament.uk/pa/ld201213/ldselect/ldpublic/140/140.pdf.

Hunter, D. (2011). Feature. *Perspectives in Public Health, 131*(3), 106-107.

Liddle, J., Gustafsson, L., Bartlett, H., & McKenna, K. (2012). Time use, role participation and life satisfaction of older people: Impact of driving status. *Australian Occupational Therapy Journal, 59,* 384-392

Member's comments. (n.d.). Cheltenham U3A. Retrieved May 22, 2014, from http://www.cheltenhamu3a.org.uk/testimonials.pdf.

Meyer, H. (2013, August 24). Older, healthier and working: Britons say no to retirement. *The Observer.* Retrieved August 30, 2013, from http://www.theguardian.com/society/2013/aug/24/working-britons-retirement.

Moore, E. (1946). Preparation for retirement. *Journal of Gerontology, 1,* 202-211.

Pettican, A., & Prior, S. (2011). 'It's a new way of life': An exploration of the occupational transition of retirement. *British Journal of Occupational Therapy, 74*(1), 12-19.

Powell, M. (2010). *The mammoth book of great British humour.* London: Robinson.

Price, C. A. (2002). Retirement for women: The impact of employment. *Journal of Women and Aging, 14*(3/4), 41-57.

Quinn, J. (2002). Changing retirement trends and their impact on elderly entitlement programs. In S. Altman & D. Schactman (Eds.), *Policies of an aging society* (p. 295). Baltimore, MD: The John Hopkins University Press.

Qureshi, H. (2012, September 29). Got a problem? Just ask Grandma. *The Guardian.* Retrieved June 25, 2014, from http://www.theguardian.com/lifeandstyle/2012/sep/29/barbara-cutie-cooper-grandmother-blogger-advice.

Shock, N. (1947). Physiological factors in development. *Review of Educational Research, 17,* 362-370.

Social Care Institute for Excellence. (2013). *Maximising the potential of reablement SCIE guide 49.* Retrieved July 4, 2013, from http://www.scie.org.uk/publications/guides/guide49/files/guide49.pdf.

U.S. Department of Health and Human Services. (2010). *Healthy People 2020*. Office of Disease Prevention and Health Promotion. Washington, DC. Retrieved from http://www.healthypeople.gov/2020/consortium/HP2020Framework.pdf.

Taylor, M., & Doverspike, D. (2003). Retirement planning and preparation. In G. Adams & T. Beehr (Eds.), *Retirement: Reasons, processes and results*. (pp. 53-82). New York, NY: Springer.

University of the Third Age. (2013). Retrieved August 30, 2013, from http://u3a.org.uk/about-u3a/history-of-u3a.html?start=1.

Williams, Z. (2012, May 19). 'Don't call us old dears. We're recycled teenagers.' *The Guardian*, p. 11.

World Health Organization. (2007). *Global age-friendly cities: A guide*. Retrieved August 30, 2013, from http://www.who.int/ageing/publications/Global_age_friendly_cities_Guide_English.pdf.

World Health Organization. (2011). *Addressing the barriers to work and employment: WHO 2011 World Report on Disability*. Retrieved July 4, 2013, from http://whqlibdoc.who.int/publications/2011/9789240685215_eng.pdf.

World Health Organization. (2012). *Good health adds life to years. Global brief for World Health Day 2012*. Retrieved August 30, 2013, from http://whqlibdoc.who.int/hq/2012/WHO_DCO_WHD_2012.2_eng.pdf.

13

Work, Legacy, and a Personal Reflection

Linda A. Hunt, PhD, OTR/L, FAOTA

You've achieved success in your field when you don't know whether what you're doing is work or play.—Warren Beatty (Martin, 2004)

A legacy is how people want to be remembered and what they leave behind for others to live by. Work ethic is a type of legacy that may be passed down by an older person to a younger person. It becomes a behavior or philosophy that is carried into the future. Legacy influences the next generation. Older people seem to give advice to future generations in line with their own approach to life (Keall, Butow, Steinhauser, & Clayton, 2011). Erikson (1982) wrote that the final stage of man's development is of *ego integrity*, the acceptance that one's life has meaning. When people believe that their lives have had meaning or purpose, then they believe they have left something of value for others to follow. This is done with the hope of improving the lives of future generations.

This book is filled with examples of ways an older person passed down a legacy of the importance of work in developing purpose in life, and how doing the very best job one can do may bring a type of happiness and contentment. There is the daughter who spoke about how her mother needed to return to part-time work because she had lost cognitive energy in full retirement and was not the same person the daughter knew. The 71-year-old mother working part-time reflected on how her daughter is a hard worker too, and has accomplishments that bring pride to the mother. She believes that she was a role model for her daughter. There is the 87-year-old office worker who does not have children, but she is a role model for others working in the office with her.

There is a beautiful documentary film called *Jiro Dreams of Sushi* (2011) that focuses on work as a legacy. The film profiles an 85-year-old sushi master and owner of Sukiyabashi Jiro, a Michelin three-star restaurant. Jiro shares his philosophy about work and what he hopes to pass on to his two sons:

> *Once you decide on your career, you must immerse yourself in it. You have to fall in love with your work. Never complain about your job. You must dedicate your life to mastering your skill. That is the secret of success, and is the key to being regarded honorably. While I*

Hunt LA, Wolverson C.
Work and the Older Person: Increasing Longevity and Well-Being (pp 147-150).
© 2015 SLACK Incorporated.

am making sushi I feel victorious. If I don't keep working, my body will become worthless. If my body stops functioning, then I have to quit. Or if I look too hideous to be here, then I will retire. It's not up to me. If the customers see me and think that I look too senile. If I stopped working at 85, I would be bored out of my mind. I would be kicked out the house. My family would kick me out for being such a nuisance. I have been able to carry on with the same job for 75 years. It's hard to slow down. I guess I'm in the last stretch of the race. I want both of my sons to continue on. They both are doing what I taught them. They will run their own restaurants. I will admit I trained my sons more strictly than the other apprentices, but I did so for the sake of their future, not because I wanted to be mean to them. It's something that I thought about from the beginning. Even if I were to be gone right now, I know they can go on. Yoshikazu [the oldest son] just needs to keep it up for the rest of his life. That's what is most important. He should just keep doing the same thing for the rest of his life.

Yoshikazu responds:

Always look ahead and above yourself. Always try to improve on yourself. Always strive to elevate your craft. That's what he taught me.

All these examples point to work as a means of purpose, reflecting the Purposeful Theory of Aging explained in Chapter 2. Growing up as a female in the 1950s provided a unique perspective on career choice, work, and trying to find purpose outside my family life. The only women I knew that worked were sales people, nurses, teachers, and office personnel. Of course, there were also women writers and entertainers. Thinking about these work choices seemed to rule everything out. I liked the idea of teaching; however, I was not attracted to working with children or being in an environment with the same people all the time. Of course, as an avid reader, there were dreams of being a writer, of being an English professor. This took education. I understood the value of education early in life. My mother would point out to me that all the successful people she knew went to college. She always voiced her own wish that she had gone to college. Because she was my role model, I knew that going to college would be a goal of mine.

When my dad lost his business, my mom went to work to help support the family. She complained about how hard it was to manage the house and work, yet she took pride in her work and it became a focus in her life. She worked for the Missouri Job Service, providing employment for people. Growing up, I saw how her employment brought better quality of life to our family. I understood that she was helping other people gain better quality of life through assisting them in securing employment. I learned that working and having an income gave one opportunities to buy and do what one wanted. Having earned income was liberating; it provided choice. I also saw the relationship between income and education. Consequently, I got my first job the day I turned 16, so I could save up for college. That was a ticket to freedom. Although I struggled with a career choice, I eventually became an occupational therapist. I continued to value how education would increase my work opportunities. I embraced the long road to earning a PhD and became a university professor, not an English professor, but a professor in occupational therapy, a profession that promotes purposeful living. What a great fit for someone who values work.

My mother's legacy taught me that I could have whatever life I wanted, as long as I worked for it. She believed that financial freedom brought freedom in other areas. This gave me a sense of responsibility and self-determination, and I knew to never blame others for problems. Ultimately, the choices were mine. I knew to show up on time, give my best effort, look for ways to improve something at work, and complete work to the best of my ability. I also learned to work with integrity and to bring that integrity to the work setting. She would tell me stories about situations at work that were challenging. I saw her cope with these difficulties, and from her examples, I learned how to continue working when my own workplace became stressful. I asked my own daughter how she viewed this work ethic legacy because I wondered if I was leaving the same legacy as my mom left me. She told me, "It has been inspiring to watch you pursue your passions and dreams through your work and education achievements. Plus, you are still the best mom a person could have."

Here is another daughter reflecting on what her mother taught her about work. Her mother's story is in Chapter 12:

For much of my life, my mom was the primary wage earner in our family, but she also worked because she enjoyed working. She taught my sisters and me independence and how to take care of ourselves and contribute to our house management! I saw her hard work earn her the respect of her coworkers and watched her receive promotions and take on more responsibility. Mom was the very best role model for work. In the banking world, it was never enough to just learn how to do a job, you had to educate yourself continuously and be part of the innovation, every day. There are continual changes in regulations and procedures in banking, so she had to always be educating herself and her staff on those changes. She has a very high standard for her work (even when she knits if it is not just right she rips the whole work apart and starts again), and expects those around her to be as dedicated and thorough. She also taught me that it is not enough to work hard and do a good job but that you should enjoy your work, or at least find a way to enjoy what you do. She derived the most pleasure from working with her customers; she was very dedicated to them. I think she stayed with her job so long because she loved working with people and she enjoyed knowing she was helpful to them. I find inspiration in her work ethic every day. Even when work is not going well, I persevere and find ways to enjoy my work. I know she is proud of the work I do, as I have always been proud of the work she did.

The following is another narrative from a granddaughter about the legacy her grandfather gave her.

Mr. Brown grew up in rural Arkansas on a small farm. To pay for tuition for a business course, Mr. Brown took out a student loan at the First National Bank in Wynne, Arkansas. He took a job at the bank while completing his studies. He performed all kinds of duties at the bank, and in 1965 became the bank president. He was Chairman of the Board from 1991 through 1996, when he retired. He still has an office as a consultant and states that he enjoys "true banking hours." Mr. Brown's legacy is that through hard work and determination, one can achieve that American dream. The desire to better himself gave him the character to love and respect his community. He made the community a better place. Megan Kelly, age 30 is Mr. Brown's granddaughter. She has early childhood memories of visiting her grandparents in Wynne, Arkansas. Her earliest observations were:

My grandpa knew everyone due to his involvement at church, [in his] community, and work. "It's a Wonderful Life" is how my dad views my grandfather. He always made positive impacts on people's lives working at the bank. He was president of the bank. Now at 92 years old, he still goes to the bank every day. His routine is to go every morning. Grandmother became sick and that took him away from work for a while. She died last year. People at the bank are his friends; they have been friends forever. He understands the value of occupying his time.

How did your grandfather influence you growing up?

Inheritance of work ethic. Strong bank ethic. Very frugal. I value being financially responsible. I admired my grandfather being self-made.

How does your grandfather's commitment to work at age 92 continue to inspire you?

Inspired me to want to stay active and involved. If you love your work, you do not want to retire. It makes me value small businesses and the community effect of that. He is so respected at 92 that the bank is willing to hold a space for him. I now understand how difficult it must be to retire. I know that he believes work has kept him sharp. Work energizes him. I also believe he gained longevity by doing something he thought was good, breathing life into others through his work. My grandmother was also a model of purposeful living. She died at 80, volunteered at the hospital gift shop till age 80. I hope to continue to create purposeful living through my career, community activities, building a family, and creating traditions around the holidays. I feel what I bring to the world will impact others positively. I don't think I will retire.

It seems that your grandfather gave you a legacy of wanting to work hard, make it on your own, and to build community. How would you describe your generation's view of the value of work?

Things have changed in that people of my generation do not value community. They do not put time into relationships to build a community and build a work environment. A lot of us are isolated due to the ability to find resources on our own. Not into mentorship as much.

Engagement in work or volunteerism has a unique attribute. In life, everyone starts out as no one. Through a life dedicated to work, volunteering, and family, one becomes a person worthy of respect. Working becomes more than providing and material gain. It becomes an identity, citizenship, and a way of living that is passed on to future generations.

It is our hope that this book inspires others' gratitude for work. We wish that those individuals who want to work or volunteer into old age achieve that goal. Take joy in living a life of purpose through occupation. Employment, like other purposeful activities, connects us with other human beings, contributes to the nature and purpose of existence, and helps develop personal well-being and personal development.

References

Erikson, E. H. (1982). *The life cycle completed*. New York, NY: Norton.

Keall, R. M., Butow, P. N., Steinhauser, K. E., & Clayton, J. M. (2011). Discussing life story, forgiveness, heritage, and legacy with patients with life-limiting illnesses. *International Journal of Palliative Nursing, 17,* 454-460.

Martin, W. P. (2004). *The best liberal quotes ever: why the left is right*. Naperville, IL: Sourcebooks.

Financial Disclosures

Dr. Ross Andel has no financial or proprietary interest in the materials presented herein.

Dr. Marian Arbesman was a consultant for the AOTA's Evidence-Based Literature Review Project.

Dr. Jane Cronin-Davis has no financial or proprietary interest in the materials presented herein.

Dr. Laura Dimmler has no financial or proprietary interest in the materials presented herein.

Erin E. Hunt has no financial or proprietary interest in the materials presented herein.

Dr. Linda A. Hunt has no financial or proprietary interest in the materials presented herein.

Dr. Nancy E. Krusen has no financial or proprietary interest in the materials presented herein.

Dr. Susan Magasi has no financial or proprietary interest in the materials presented herein.

Dr. Denise M. Nepveux has not disclosed any relevant financial relationships.

Dr. Jeff Snodgrass has not disclosed any relevant financial relationships.

Aimée Thompson has not disclosed any relevant financial relationships.

Caroline Wolverson has no financial or proprietary interest in the materials presented herein.

Michael Wolverson has not disclosed any relevant financial relationships.

Index

3